Tenderly Lift Me

Literature and Medicine
MARTIN KOHN AND CAROL DONLEY, EDITORS

1. *Literature and Aging: An Anthology*
   EDITED BY MARTIN KOHN, CAROL DONLEY, AND DELESE WEAR

2. *The Tyranny of the Normal: An Anthology*
   EDITED BY CAROL DONLEY AND SHERYL BUCKLEY

3. *What's Normal? Narratives of Mental and Emotional Disorders*
   EDITED BY CAROL DONLEY AND SHERYL BUCKLEY

4. *Recognitions: Doctors and Their Stories*
   EDITED BY CAROL DONLEY AND MARTIN KOHN

5. *Chekhov's Doctors: A Collection of Chekhov's Medical Tales*
   EDITED BY JACK COULEHAN

6. *Tenderly Lift Me: Nurses Honored, Celebrated, and Remembered*
   BY JEANNE BRYNER

Tenderly Lift Me

Nurses Honored, Celebrated, and Remembered

❧

Jeanne Bryner

❧

The Kent State University Press

KENT & LONDON

❧

© 2004 by The Kent State University Press, Kent, Ohio 44242

ALL RIGHTS RESERVED

Library of Congress Catalog Card Number 2003021420

ISBN 0-87338-802-X

Manufactured in the United States of America

08 07 06 05 04   5 4 3 2 1

LIBRARY OF CONGRESS CATALOGING-IN-PUBLICATION DATA

Bryner, Jeanne, 1951–

Tenderly lift me : nurses honored, celebrated, and remembered / Jeanne Bryner.

p. cm.

Includes bibliographical references.

ISBN 0-87338-802-X (pbk. : alk. paper) ∞

1. Nurse and patient—Poetry.   2. Nursing—poetry.   3. Nurses—Poetry.

4. Nurse and patient.   5. Nursing.   6. Nurses.   I. Title.

PS3552.R995T46 2004   811'.54—dc22   2003021420

British Library Cataloging-in-Publication data are available.

For my mother who wanted
to give me ballet lessons.
It's all right, mom;
this is the way I dance.

When they were ill, I mourned before the Lord
in sackcloth, asking him to make them well.

PSALMS 35:13

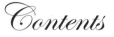

Contents

Preface and Acknowledgments   xi

Introduction *by Suzanne Poirier and Rosemary Field*   xvi

Part 1

Learning the Body   3

Standing There   4

Side Rails   5

Father Damien   6

    To the Place of Orchids   7

Rose Hawthorne Lathrop   9

    Covering Lilacs   11

Sister Elizabeth Kenny   13

    Elsewhere Sparrows: A Note to Some Physicians   14

Rita Marie Magdaleno   16

    Teaching Women to Speak   17

Part 2

Sandi Petek   21

    Village   23

Carlyann Markusic   25

    Story   26

Sue Zenko   29

    What Has Happened   31

Joanne Fowler   33

    One Nurse's Job: Eye Recovery on a Kindergartner   34

Rita Richards   36

    Testimony   37

Pat Austin   39

    A Boat They Float In   40

Elfriede Anton 43
    Underground: A Note to My Brother, Kurt 45
Theresa Marcotte Kokrak 46
    To Save What We Most Love 47
Terri Swearingen 49
    The Evolution of Light: East Liverpool, Ohio, Site of the
        WTI Incinerator 50
Helen Albert 52
    Juba 53
Esther Baker 55
    Letter to Josephine, 1996 57

Part 3

Renaissance Sketchbook: A Woman's Story 61
Miscarriage: The Nurse Speaks to the Baby 62
Maude Callen 63
    For Maude Callen: Nurse Midwife, Pineville, South Carolina, 1951 64
    Holding Back the World 65
Helen Troy 66
    Letter to Christine: Girl Baby Found, Ohio Hospital, 1958 67
Sylvia Engelhardt 69
    How I Lost My Job as a Staff Nurse in 1969, Because
        I Was Pregnant 70
    August Delivery 71

Part 4

Hope Chest: What the Heart Teaches 75
Carol L. Johnson 77
    On My Gloves Blood Dries in a Pattern Like Faded
        Roses in Wallpaper 78
    At Dusk, Two Women Trace a Heart's River 79
Jeannette Price 81
    Letter to World War I Surgeon Dr. Henry Russell, from
        Nurse Jeanette Price, September 1929 83

Part 5

Nora Mary Carmody McNicholas 87
    What It Cost to Cross the Atlantic 88

Jeanne Bryner   90
  Becoming a Nurse   91
  Breathless   92
  Body of Knowledge: Remembering Diploma Nursing Schools, 1976   92
  Letter from Ward Three   94
Avanell Arlene Sutherland   96
  Loving Women   98
  This Red Oozing   98
  The Labor of Tenderness   100
  After the Battle: In a Room Where We Have Tried to Save a Life   101

Part 6

Butterfly   105
Genevieve Schmitt   107
  Mentally Traumatized Unit: Nursing Assignment, England 1942   109
Phyllis Fischer   110
  *To My Town Came a Snow Storm, Nurse's Diary, City Hospital
    of Cleveland, Ohio, November 24, 1950*   111
Rebecca Ann Needham Anderson   114
  Call and Response   115
  Birch Canoe   116
Betty Jane Panchik   117
  November 1963   118
Hortense Wood   120
  At Thirteen, I Decide to Become a Nurse   121
  Warblers   123
Jane Ball   124
  What Nurses Do: The Marriage of Suffering and Healing   125
June Elizabeth Conolly   127
  School Nurse   128
Helen Krier   130
  Christmas Is Another Moon   132
Darrell Grace   133
  When I Tell My Mother I Want to Be a Doctor   134
Judy Waid   136
  Pentimento   138
Lynda Arnold   140
  Begin Again   142

Part 7

The Sisters of St. Joseph's Hospitallers   147
    Interview with Sister Denis of St. Joseph's Hospitallers
       Colony of Montreal, New France, 1694   148
Kate Cumming   151
    Wait for Morning: From Kate Cumming's Journal   152
Jane Stuart Woolsey   155
    Jane Stuart Woolsey, Union Nurse from Camp, near
       Alexandria, 1862   157
    Nurse's Letter, May 30, 1864, Armory Square Hospital, WDC 157
Rebecca Taylor   159
    A Tribute to Miss Rebecca Taylor upon Retirement after
       Thirty-Four Years   160
Edith Cavell   162
    Houses Are Burning: Belgium, 1915   163

Part 8

If It Weren't For Ears   169
The Brain's Soliloquy   170
Clay Pigeon   172
In Praise of Hands   173

Permissions   175
Notes on the Text   177
Bibliography   179

Preface and Acknowledgments

Imagine a circle the size of a dinner plate. It can be china or paper or plastic. Now, say to yourself, "This circle represents my life." Take a crayon, any color, and shade in the parts of the circle that represent your work: the alarm ringing, a uniform being pressed, the appointment card taped to the counter, the coffee mug wedged inside your car door, your plastic card opening the parking lot gate, the sameness of beige lockers, the push and pull of responsibilities, joys and frustrations as you move through another shift, the drive home where you catalog wins and losses, and the hard sound all keys make when they strike a table. You might ask yourself if you are the warden or the prisoner. And perhaps, on any given day, you are both. Still, this is your life, and it deserves to be honored and celebrated.

I am a nurse, and, looking back, I believe I have been a nurse my entire life, though I've only been licensed to practice since 1979. I am an apprentice poet who was inspired by two poets and their use of language: Chris Llewellyn in *Fragments from the Fire* and Dolores Kendrick in *The Women of Plums*. Llewellyn's retelling of the Triangle Shirtwaist Factory fire and Kendrick's slave narratives shaped into poetry were the catalyst for this manuscript about historical and contemporary nurses. These two women have been beacons for my incredible journey of research and interviews, and I thank them.

There will never be enough books about women and the part of their circle that illustrates work. There will never be enough books to praise the lives of nurses. Because I have the gift of a college education and an understanding partner, I can steal the weeks and years I need to tell my stories about being a woman, a wife, a mother, and a nurse. Many of my sisters cannot. Women comprise two thirds of the world's illiterate population. And so my sense of urgency, my need to speak, is the tin cup I drag across bars every day, begging to be heard.

Being a thief, I have no shame. My interviewer's questions and pen have pried open memory's door for others and myself. The past is not always a friendly country, but it is here we uncover the truth of our lives. I do not apologize for taking years to finish what remain several pale handprints retrieved for each nurse's life. An entire biography is incapable of capturing the bend and heave of a person's dreams and hungers, nightmares and prayers, so these sculpted vignettes are like hurried notes I've written to the world.

Like anyone who has served under pressure, I have an aching to stop and an aching to continue writing this book; however, two nurses in this collection will never witness another spring. Time is always the enemy. Genevieve Schmitt and Nora McNicholas, ages ninety-four and ninety-two, died before this book was accepted for publication. I'm sad because they will never hold the book, but I rejoice that the book somehow holds them—two violets pressed by the dew of ninety-plus summers. Being nurses, they knew the body is like a train; it must travel as long as there's fire in the engine; a person cannot stick her foot out to slow the train or to keep it from going where it's bound.

Helen Albert and Esther Baker have suffered strokes in the last three years: Helen is in a wheelchair; all her mental faculties are intact; Esther has made a fine recovery with minimal memory problems. Carlyann Markusic has had eye surgery and is now battling a blood disorder. Hortense Wood has completed her BSN.

And I have read many, many books surrounding my subject matter, even one about passenger pigeons, which are now extinct. What do birds have in common with nurses? When passenger pigeons lived, people hunted them, trapped them, sewed their eyes shut and strapped them to tree branches to lure other pigeons to their death. Hunters would not listen to naturalists who said, "One day they will disappear." It seemed impossible because during migration season, skies darkened from the flocks, like an eclipse. Think about all the closed nursing schools and how many fine nurses we lose annually to burnout, illness, and retirement. Globally and daily, people who are not nurses are trained to *give bedside care.* This practice is subtle and deliberate; it can be dangerous; it has the potential for elimination.

I want people to care about nurses the way nurses care about people who are total strangers—folks who have been so ill they have no memory of surgery or their stays in emergency rooms and intensive care units. Nurses are human and sometimes a little heroic, but not from heaven. For a moment, I want you, dear reader, to imagine your next operation and recovery without the nurse's voice above your bed. Negative space can be frightening, and nurses are educated professionals who struggle for autonomy. Let every silence become a journal page. I want our life stories lifted and written, microfilmed and stored like our patients' charts. These stories deserve to be studied in universities, read in high schools and introduced in kindergartens. To protect nurses and their vital work of patient advocacy, I want congress members and senators to pass appropriate legislation. Retired nurses should be able to purchase medications, take vacations, and pay their utilities. When readers finish this book, I want them to find a nurse and say, "Thank you."

To all the women who granted interviews and trusted me with their extraordinary stories, I am grateful. They made sandwiches for me, baked cookies, and met me at odd hours to eat pancakes and bagels and Chinese food. I stayed in their homes, shadowed them on the job and asked them to walk barefoot on broken glass, because that is the floor in the house of memory. They are women with great courage and character. They are who I want to be when I grow up. My friend Rita Magdaleno wisely suggested I get photos of the nurses as I interviewed them. Because I believe the face tells an important layer of the life story, I asked permission for photographs. Most of the women agreed, but I respected the decision of two nurses who declined photographs.

To write such a thoughtful introduction, Dr. Suzanne Poirier and Rosemary Field dedicated an enormous amount of time reading and processing this manuscript. My pen fails me when I try to compensate such labor with language. They know me only through my words, and I them through theirs. We have never met in person, yet I feel they are my sisters.

I wish to acknowledge the many people who have helped me become a better thinker, creative writer, and person. Many of these poems were written in fulfillment of my senior thesis in the honors college of Kent State University. My thesis director, who became also my mentor and friend, was Maggie Anderson; her poetry workshops opened new worlds for my writing life. Through her classroom assignments, my first historical poems were born. I am grateful for her common sense, scholarship, and friendship. I received early encouragement for writing from the following professors: Elizabeth Hoobler, Gloria Young, and Vivian Pemberton; I thank them for suggesting books and sending me back to the piano bench over and over until the music was just right.

I am indebted to the following people and organizations whose generosity has helped my writing grow and mature: the Wick Poetry Program at Kent State University for awarding me scholarships and selecting my chapbook, *Breathless*, for publication in 1995; Bucknell University for granting me the 1992 Fellowship for Younger Poets; the Associated Writing Program (AWP) for giving me its 1992 Intro Award; and the Ohio Arts Council for the 1997 Ohio Arts Individual Artist Fellowship. I thank Walter Wick and Robert Wick for generously supporting poetry through their Kent State University foundation, Jack Stadler for supporting poetry at Bucknell University, and the AWP for encouraging young writers with the Intro Awards. When I received the Ohio Arts Council Fellowship, Forum Health Trumbull Memorial Hospital granted me a sabbatical for travel and research interviews. I thank the Ohio Arts Council for their vote of confidence and my former director of nursing, Lois McLean, for understanding the importance of this project.

Two groups of artists adapted several of these poems for stage. The northeastern Ohio collaborative worked together for two-and-a-half years performing *Lift*,

Breathe, Carry: Life and Art in Three Movements in Texas, West Virginia, Kentucky, New York, and Ohio. Artists in the Ohio collaborative were Zen Campbell, Emmy Krielkamp, Lisa Craze, Nolan O'Dell, Renee Reinhart, Randy Niemi, Linda Kahn, Keith Newman, Charity Herb, and Melissa Wintringham. Under the direction of Nicole Pearce at the California Institute of the Arts, the artists who performed, designed, and created for *Childhood's End* were Kim Bennink, Jillian Frost, Amantha May, Frances Hearn, Heather Hartruft, Jeanette Scherrer, Leah Mercer, Kathleen Reese, Julie Giroux, Anna Pasquale, Wren Crosley, Ashley Nason, and Dana Vasquez-Eberhardt. Both of these groups dedicated heart and soul to the performances. It was a privilege to be part of the northeastern Ohio group, and I learned a great deal about theater, friendship, and the development of both. Each performance was unique and breathtaking; I can never thank the artists enough for all their hard work.

Few books are born without the sweat of research. Librarians and archivists at many libraries have assisted me over the past six-and-a-half years, and I would like to thank Sr. Nicole Bussieres, RHSJ, in Montreal; Martha Stone at the Treadwell Library at Massachusetts General Hospital, Boston; Jack Eckert of the Francis A. Countway Library of Medicine at Harvard, Cambridge; Jane Brown, curator of the Waring Historical Library at the Medical University of South Carolina, Charleston; Alex Rankin, nursing archivist at Boston University; Stephen E. Novak, head of Archives and Special Collections, Columbia University, New York; Caryn Kish, archivist, Sisters of Charity of St. Augustine, Cleveland; and Martha Marie Eduard, OP, Dominican Sisters, New York. Several librarians at the Newton Falls Public Library have also been very helpful; special thanks to Brenda Charney, Barbara Jones, Holly Ryan, Laura Alldridge, Debbie Augusta, and Darlene MacKenzie.

Realizing the historical importance of labor documentation, John Russo and Sherry Linkon, codirectors of the Center for Working Class Studies at Youngstown State University, facilitated the transcribing and archiving of my interview tapes, which may be studied by scholars in the future. For the work of their lives and offering to preserve these oral histories, I thank them. I am indebted to the Ford Foundation for their support of the Center for Working Class Studies.

A very special thanks to Doris Needham, mother of Rebecca Anderson, for sharing photographs and biographical information. Also, special thanks to the family of Arlene Sutherland for participating in a communal interview and sharing stories and photographs. For trusting me with her Aunt Jenny's World War I photo album, mess kit, canteen, and plate, I especially thank Esther Gundry.

Many individuals read and reread these poems during their long evolution. I thank my sisters, Nancy Henderson and Mary Kay Martindale, for always reading the *new* ones and giving feedback. My dear friend Diane Fisher has also been a faithful reader, guiding the development of so many stories. My daughter, Summar, worked hours and hours of her computer magic to get bios and poems into separate files; I appreciate all her efforts. Finally, always and forever, I thank my best friend and partner, David, for reading the entire manuscript and commenting honestly on it and for suffering my absences as I worked.

I gratefully acknowledge several publications in which many of the poems originally appeared in earlier forms.

Appalachian Heritage 30.2 (Spring 2002): "Loving Women" and "Hope Chest: What the Heart Teaches."

Breathless, by Jeanne Bryner (Kent, Ohio: Kent State University Press, 1995): "Maude Callen, Nurse Midwife, Pineville, South Carolina, 1951" and "Breathless."

Hawaii Review 21.3 (Summer/Fall 1998): "Becoming a Nurse."

The HeART of Nursing: Expressions of Creative Arts in Nursing, ed. M. Cecelia Wendler (Indianapolis: Center Nursing Publishing Press, 2002): "After the Battle: In a Room Where We Have Tried to Save a Life."

International Journal of Arts Medicine 5, no. 2 (1997): "In Praise of Hands."

POEM 80 (1998): "To the Place of Orchids."

Poetry East 37–38 (Spring 1994): "Butterfly."

Prairie Schooner 68.2 (1994): "Letter from Ward Three."

This Time, This Place (Cleveland: Poets' League of Greater Cleveland, 1996) "Interview with Sister Denis of St. Joseph's Hospitallers, Colony of Montreal, New France, 1694."

West Branch 44 (1999): "Miscarriage: The Nurse Speaks to the Baby."

Introduction

SUZANNE POIRIER AND ROSEMARY FIELD

From Florence Nightingale, of Victorian England and the battlefields of the Crimean War, to Carol Hathaway, of the contemporary television program *ER* and the battlefield of the inner-city Chicago emergency room, nurses have often been perceived as "angels of mercy," bastions of compassion and heroism. Along the way, Charles Dickens's Sairy Gamp and Ken Kesey's Nurse Ratched have painted an opposing image of nurses as cruel, selfish, and morally suspect. For good measure, there are the countless greeting cards and cartoons that picture a buxom, usually blonde, bombshell in a tight, short, white dress standing provocatively over a scantily gowned, bandaged, usually male patient. None of these images are of ordinary women dealing with people daily for years on end. Certainly, there are nurses who are heroic, cruel, or (maybe even) sexual sirens, but these are extreme portraits—or portraits of nurses in extreme, often fleeting moments. Over the course of their careers, nurses may inspire, frighten, comfort, arouse, save, or even harm patients. They are probably many different things to many different people. And these people are many different things to each nurse, often inextricable from the moments of her or his own constantly changing life.

In *Tenderly Lift Me* Jeanne Bryner corrects such public stereotyping and ignorance. She brings us the daily lives of real nurses, past and present. Her poems immerse us in the sights, smells, textures, and sounds of nurses' immediate, physical work with people dying, living, and struggling to live. She shows us that nurses are as human and vulnerable as the patients they serve, at the same time that they struggle with their own vulnerability so that they may succeed in being what patients need them to be. At times they embrace this challenge, but at times they flee it. Often they return, but sometimes they do not. Bryner presents three kinds of portraits in this collection: those of widely known, historical figures; those of nurses from across her home state of Ohio; and those from the voice of Bryner's own nursing experience. Together, these poems demonstrate that nurses' work cannot be captured or contained in frozen, one-dimensional, and exaggerated images. They also demonstrate that nurses' work involves—above subservience and mechanistic repetition—imagination, resolve, adaptability, and leadership. Compassion and caring, placed in this more complex constellation of qualities, become an end achieved through determination, self-examination, open-mindedness, and love.

We read and discussed the poems in this collection from two different perspectives: the first, of a nurse of twenty years and the second, of a literature and feminist studies teacher for an equal number of years. During this exercise we roamed in the nature of nursing as well as that of poetry, and in the history of nursing in particular and of women in general. Although this introduction is a creation of that collaboration, let us also introduce ourselves to you individually here, briefly, and tell you what we each brought to this conversation.

ROSEMARY FIELD:

It has been twenty years since I graduated from nursing school. I still remember my sense of bewilderment as I launched myself into what I thought then was a noble, pristine career: I would help people, take care of them during their most vulnerable time. I would provide a service to the sick and dying, and I would be able to make them better. I would make my parents proud. I would leave the profession a better place. I was full of ideas of what I could do for the individuals I would care for and the profession I would commit to. Twenty years after graduation, I remain committed to my work with the same sense of awe I had when I started; however, now I understand why. The reasons are clearer now. The care I provide my patients and my colleagues makes a difference despite the sometimes-invisible nature of my work—in that sense I am, paradoxically, a powerful influence. Bryner's poems brought to me a kaleidoscope of images that I related to in my personal journey as a nurse. I realized that as nurses we are not all that different. Despite the diversity in clinical settings, roles, and experiences, we are all connected, and it is in that connection that we influence each other's lives. We are drawn together by the sacred and profane nature of our work, by the struggle we all have to find meaning in our work, and by the sense of both the exhaustion and the exhilaration we experience as we put our education into action, however unique each of us is. For me, the poems in *Tenderly Lift Me* provide vivid images of nurses doing their work. They describe the varied settings of our work, the transformation of our work as a function of the passage of time, and the personal growth nurses experience as we engage or integrate our work into our lives. The poems describe the people we are—the people we bring to work with us.

SUZANNE POIRIER:

Literature brings people's lives before us. Poetry can distill the essence of a life into a haunting phrase or striking image. Feminism has taught me to look for the too often *overlooked* contributions women have made to the world. For me, Bryner's poetry captures the strengths of both literature's ability to make us see our world anew and feminism's desire to celebrate the heroic, triumphant, and tragic in everyday life. The poems show us young girls (with one exception, all the nurses depicted here are women) deciding—and sometimes being directed—to become nurses. We see nurses subordinating their own lives, sometimes willingly but sometimes reluctantly, to the demands of their work and the expectations of others. Yet the meaning and power of that work often subverts or transcends that subordination. These nurses often describe their work in the words and images of wife, mother, housekeeper, and sexual partner. All of these nurses' professional identities are inseparable from their understanding of themselves as women in a world that is often hostile to them but that also often values the comfort and compassion it associates with women. All these factors can create tremendous tension within each nurse's life, and we hear these women at times protesting and at other times finding their own comfort in this warp and woof that makes the tapestry of a nurse's life.

As we explored these poems together, we were struck probably above all with the very *unheroic* way most of these nurses portrayed what was often, to us, very heroic work. Lives are lived in the daily acts that necessity calls for. Even in her portraits of historical nurses, Bryner gives us the homely details that make work meaningful to nursing pioneers. "All night, hold people // close, children, foul persons," says Florence Nightingale in "Learning the Body," speaking of a simple deed made perhaps less simple by its circumstances. Bryner anoints Father Damien as a nurse in her poem about his work, "To the Place of Orchids." Sent to care for the lepers on a lush island in Hawaii, the only lushness before his eyes appears in the decay of human bodies:

> The sea was behind me, and I changed,
> years of bandages glistening with sap,
> taken down every day like wires from their
> limbs, sweet bodies ripening, rotting,
> like pieces of fruit in a bowl, and me,
> trembling under God's white, white clouds.

Sent to this place in response to his request to serve others, Father Damien had not reckoned on the human devastation he would encounter or its effect on him, a beautiful despair that Bryner represents in likening bodies to ripe fruit that goes on to putrefy. This normal course of vegetable nature seemed to him a cruel, unjust fate for people whom God made "in His own image." Bryner depicts Father Damien as constantly taunted by this inevitability because he had always believed that service meant making people whole again.

History may record Father Damien and Florence Nightingale as heroes who triumphed against all odds, a triumph that proved their mettle, endurance, and brilliance, but Bryner's images of the torture of ripe and rotting bodies and "foul persons" who must be held through the night are, for her, the true measures of these people's heroism. She writes in "Standing There" that nurses' true accounts are histories neither "of healers / dressed in . . . halo caps" nor of magical healers "chanting blue power" nor of influential persuaders who pound "a fist against mahogany conference tables." Instead, those histories are written in moments of fear and uncertainty, "when pain was thunder / and we waited, worked in a world of raw light / so bright its camera blinded."

And it is these moments that all nurses share, moments recorded in the poems that unite history's remembered heroes and the unsung heroes of every city's hospitals and clinics. The prevailing image of nurses in all these poems— whether at war, in the school nurse's office, in exotic lands, or in the hospital— is one of work. As we read and discussed the poems in this collection, though, we also identified several themes that cut across the sections Bryner creates here. Those themes, in no particular order, are 1) the decision to be a nurse, 2) the journey of becoming a nurse, 3) the disillusionments in nursing, 4) the hard or ugly truths that nurses must learn, and 5) the affirmations of nursing. These categories often overlap, a further testimony to the ever-evolving experience of a nurse's professional and personal life. Moreover, the poems in all these categories are always, primarily, about patients and the other people who have influenced these nurses. From these poems, we see that nursing is, ultimately, about each nurse's relationships with all the people she or he meets.

The decision to become a nurse is often made early, according to the stories told here. Sometimes it is based on an experience with illness early in life, but other times it is based on less inspired circumstances, such as limited economic and professional opportunities for women at the time or even the desire to stay with a friend who has chosen to study nursing. Sometimes it is a combination of practicality and passion. For Hortense Wood ("At Thirteen, I Decide to Become a Nurse"), thirteen years old, with "the legs of a colt and the breasts / of a sparrow," appendicitis was a terrifying affliction. It brought her, for the first time, naked and in pain, under the "clumsy fingers" of the "pale hands" of the white doctor who ordered her to "'lie still and flat; make your tummy soft.'" In this world of whiteness—both the hospital and her doctor—she felt alone in a strange land, sleeping "under sheets her Mama didn't wash." But the nurses, although they were probably mostly white as well, were not so foreign (or as frightening). Moving quietly and constantly through the hospital, they were a refuge, "churches with their doors thrown open." Their "dresses sewn of snow" and their "faces of Mary" offered refuge—and perhaps a familiar comfort in their resemblance to the women of the Mothers' Board, who are beneficent guardians in traditional African American church services. It was these nurses who drew her. Who were they? What did they do? Hortense heard two answers, both of which led her to choose this career: "Mama said *angels of mercy;* / Daddy said *pride.*" Bryner's imagery of the work of Nurse Wood years later conveys this undiminished sense of both pride and mercy through the work of her nursing. Flaking skin becomes "snowflakes . . . born in old men's socks"; and "grannies trade stories" for "extra pudding," stories that take the nurse back in time to the lives of her patients before their illness, old age, or death.

Bryner's use of simple images and plain language to evoke a highly emotional experience appears even in the titles of her poems, such as the one about Carol Johnson, a cardiothoracic nurse practitioner: "On My Gloves Blood Dries in a Pattern Like Faded Roses in Wallpaper." This is a poem about the journey to become a nurse. We see Carol as she has reached the level of a technically skilled surgical nurse who works in the operating room as a partner to the surgeon in complicated heart surgery. She "harvest[s] saphenous veins," cutting from her patient's thigh the vein that the surgeon will use to replace diseased arteries in the heart. Bryner again uses religious imagery, as the nurse "cut[s] the fresh / Wafer" of vein, offering it up to the heart. The nurse offers up to the surgeon, in a ritual of subservience couched in an image of ordinary housework—"Wipe with red dishrags, nurses' work never done"—that avoids being demeaning because the nurse's skill is as beautiful and mysterious as the surgeon's. Her gesture, however, is more personal and soothing. The nurse's curved needle becomes a "half-moon" that stitches a "secret embroidery," and "clos[ing]" (another surgical chore) is offered as a way to "comfort the leg oozing, mourning its loss." To the nurse, this leg is as precious and as necessary as the heart itself, and the leg's blood on her gloves evokes memories of old-fashioned wallpaper, whose rich floral pattern one might find in an old-fashioned grandmother's quiet, dimmed front parlor. The nurse, however advanced in her art, still manages to engage in, as Rosemary has said, both "the sacred and profane."

This journey has brought Carol Johnson to a place of pride in highly technical work that she still sees as providing comfort to her patient. That comfort has not been overwhelmed by the sterility of the operating room or the mechanical precision of the tasks she performs. Other poems, however, show the often-rocky road that nurses travel before they (hopefully) reach this balance of technique and compassion. The "oozing" leg in this poem evokes compassion for a part of the patient's body that is often trivialized in the larger picture of cardiac surgery. "This Red Oozing" brings us into the emergency room and reminds us that the usual fare of the ER is far from usual for the patients who come there. In this poem, the nurse speaks to a rape victim in a personal tone that counters the "*I-told-you-so eyes*" of the sheriff and the physicians who "speak like priests" as they do the standard rape exam. Such attitudes transform the woman's personal horror and the rapist's brutality into clinical evidence: "trying / to mount rage on slides." The nurse accepts the horror of this story, even though she feels she knows it already—"we hear it / nearly every week." And she knows, too, that these events are not routine for this woman—or any woman. She speaks about the victimization that this woman will now suffer repeatedly, both in retelling her story countless times to physicians, police, and even friends, and in reliving the violation in every daily act of her life:

> how he rapes you
> endlessly: how he crawls out of your lipstick
> tube in the morning, slithers out of the soapy
> washcloth in the shower, snickers every Friday
> when you dust those photos on your stand.
> How his boots climb the back stairs
> of your mind year after year
> as he comes and comes and comes.

Here, the nurse makes personal what can become institutional. In doing so, she returns her patient's humanity to her in the face of the necessary acts of medical treatment. At the same time, this exercise returns to the nurse the patient's humanity—as well as the humanity of the nurse herself, who becomes vulnerable through witnessing such events.

The lessons that nurses must learn are hard, often ugly ones—like rape, AIDS, child abuse, war, abandonment. Sometimes they are too hard to survive, as we hear in the poems about disillusionment. Noticeably, the disillusionment is usually not about the work of nursing but instead about the cruelty of the world that surrounds patients—and sometimes nurses. In "What Has Happened," we meet Sue Zenko, whose polite, almost whimsical address to her nursing teacher, Miss Morley, offers a stark picture of the complex combination of work, feelings, and economics that can drive some women from nursing. Sue, who graduated first in her nursing class, has left nursing to become a "waitress in a Chinese restaurant," where she earns more in tips than she did as a nurse, and where "there are no old men peeing in wastebaskets / or young mothers bleeding from leukemia." Her images move from the humorously pathetic to the tragic to the unimaginable, as she asks Miss Morley to "[r]emember the little girl scalded in the tub / by her parents, and the broomstick // they somehow shoved up her rectum?" She tries to forget "crying in the night" from one of her first patients, but she has never completely succeeded in forgetting the career she first chose. "What has happened to your blue hair / and white gloves?" she asks Miss Morley. Is Miss Morley an anachronism who was unable to prepare Sue for the world of nursing in 1965, or has she reached an ideal level of calm, propriety, and balance in the face of a harsh world that Sue could not achieve? Was it harder for Sue to leave nursing or to feel she had failed Miss Morley— and idealistic nurses everywhere? Waitressing, whatever relief it offers, is also empty. Her achievements are mastery of the use of chopsticks and the ability to "explain every dish on the menu." She offers Miss Morley no excuses for her defection, but her empty voice suggests that she feels a loss nevertheless.

A sense of connection to other people, which characterizes most of these poems, is missing in Sue Zenko's story. Carlyann Markusic in "Story" is also feeling isolated, but through no choice of her own. She returned to her work in the emergency department sooner than she had planned after the birth of her baby: "responsibility draws its own timetable—// episiotomy healed or not— and when the rent's due." When she corrected a policeman, Joe, who was badgering her patient, Joe's "eyes / went dark and hard" and he suddenly grabbed her and pulled his gun. Blinky Spell, the wino "[t]wo beds / over," the only person who begged Joe to spare her, clung to her until other officials freed her. Carlyann refutes the adage that one's life passes before one's eyes when death threatens; instead, "I peed my pants." When she was finally rescued, all the people around her expressed concern for the stresses in Joe's life; Carlyann received no sympathy, was not allowed to go home because the shift was understaffed, and was sent to shower in the doctors' lounge and change into a clean set of scrubs. Alone in the shower,

> soap and water running hot
> down thighs to the soft place where I still bled
> from my son, I cried and cried and cried.
>
> I could see his smooth pink face
> how he was so small
> and already able to wave his fists.

Bryner has Carlyann contrast the hard imagery of her treatment by Joe and Mrs. Klemm, her supervisor, with the softness of her baby's skin and her own still raw episiotomy, a contrast that also symbolizes the nurse, who, paradoxically, is expected always to be "soft" while being in control, on her toes, unflappable—when in reality she has also to protect the soft, vulnerable core of her own self.

Still, most nurses grow from these hard lessons. Indeed, at the end of their careers, many nurses can imagine no other life for themselves. Judy Waid reached this point by carefully finding a way to nurture her "softness" through a long career of hard work in a spinal-cord rehab center. Also a painter, she speaks in her poem, "Pentimento":

> After twenty-two years,
> I make bold sweeping gestures
> as if I've earned the right to free
> what can be developed in this space.

The boldness of her artistic gesture contrasts with the restricted, often halting movements of her patients, who find their bodies contained within the small spaces defined by their disability. She paints a mother, son, and daughter climbing a hill together, running and strong and with the "desire . . . not [to] be contained"—even though they are contained within the frame of her canvas. Her painting is not so much an escape from her work as it is a recognition of the unfettered spirits of her patients. In her painting, the woman with her children holds their hands "to increase strength," an act of intimacy and connection that must occur every day in her work as a nurse. Judy restores the beauty of bodies' simple movements, perhaps memorializing the actions they once possessed or celebrating the life they are now recreating. In this way, painting incorporates her work and her art—perhaps even a visible metaphor for the art of nursing. As such, however, her painting is not a release from, but more a fuller integration of, herself with the demands of nursing. For her next painting, she moves indoors, into a warm, small cafe, where "fishermen in gray woolen caps" talk about "the efforts of daily life." Their own physically demanding work once more reminds her of the primacy of the body, but here, eating the warm soup the waitress brings her and hearing the men's voices, something magical happens. She becomes a part of the painting, herself seated among these people, and she can finally "forget / everything." In this place of quiet solitude, she can nourish herself with the peace and healing she paints for others. Through her painting, Waid finds a way to heal herself.

Throughout these poems, nurses' closeness to patients and the comfort this connection brings to both of them is often symbolized by physical touching and images of hands. In Waid's painting, the mother and children hold hands. As Bryner has Waid say, "To increase strength, I make them hold hands," a deliberate, therapeutic connection. In "Covering Lilacs," Bryner writes about Rose Hawthorne Lathrop (pioneer hospice nurse and daughter of the author Nathaniel Hawthorne), who worked with people dying from cancer with her "bare hands," scorning her era's belief that cancer was contagious. Bryner continues here also the imagery of women's domestic, everyday work to describe the often-repugnant work of Lathrop and her friend Alice. She likens hard lumps of cancer to "sugar pears" and describes soft subcutaneous tumors as "soft as grapes," and a tumor that has erupted from the skin is "opening like tulips." The women who undertake this work are more usually at home among the orchards and flowerbeds of their easy, middle-class lives. They work in well-stocked kitchens, but now they oversee a roomful of people with red eyes that "ooze, like egg yolks." Instead of a closed house or kitchen, they now leave their "door open, the way / a farmer does his barn" who grooms and makes comfortable his "lame," "winded," and "fester[ing]" horses. Again, Bryner depicts nursing in its daily acts of humaneness, her domestic imagery suggesting that this work may be ordinary in the traditional lives of women at the same time that its very necessity in this untraditional setting makes this work anything but ordinary. Rose and Alice protect their charges, covering them each day with "cotton sheets," the same way they used to "cover lilacs before the frost." This gesture of protecting fragile flowers from a killing frost, when applied to hospice work, complicates this act of gardening, as the nurses seek to protect their patients from a harsh, lonely dying. For them, the spring to come will not be an earthly one: their nurses are easing their way into an eternal rebirth.

In an era when nurses are becoming more technologically skilled, are being made more accountable for their "productivity" and their contributions to "patient outcomes," Bryner has chosen to celebrate the magical, even mystical elements of nursing that cannot be measured. This art of nursing often goes unnoticed, unrecognized. As the good nurse is an artist, Bryner uses her own art to reveal the intangible core of nursing to us. This core is universal, transcending time and place. These nurses, many of them invisible to the eyes of history—and often even to their patients and the other health professionals they work with—restore and create beauty every day, often from the most frightening, unlikely materials. In the process, they also find themselves, as nursing, at its most rewarding, is a journey of constant growth.

Part 1

I don't expect to touch the sky with my two hands.

Sappho

LEARNING THE BODY

after Florence Nightingale's Notes on Nursing

The heat of the body must be examined
by the hand from time to time.
Brush knotted hair, hold people close
at night, children, foul persons.

Be terrified of all methods, very rarely expose
the breath and bodies of the sick.
In your apron carry spoons sticky
with the sun's honey.

Guard against confusion, remember Socrates,
become the quiet pulse.
Entered in sleep men and women evaporate
into themselves, into the air.

Flesh fades, a wine-soiled dress,
every seam needs repair.
Be motionless, think this: where is the tea,
yellow lotion, and writing paper?

The little house burning down is a beggar
passing a bad night.
A door opens, it is a fever
speaking in tongues. All night, people hold

close, children, foul persons.
Learn the body in the bed, any sore,
red gauze damp as poultice,
not suddenly, not in a rush.

Say, *There was blood, I carried water.*
These are my hands. I am not Jesus.
Make the story a song.

STANDING THERE

Our history isn't an album of healers
dressed in snowy uniforms, white oxfords,
and halo caps. We do not saunter hallways
and giggle pink words.

This narrative is not about Merlin or medicine
men chanting blue power over steamy rocks,
nor is it a fist against mahogany conference tables
or the kitten's whimper in a rainstorm.

Our logbooks record moments when pain was thunder
and we waited, worked in a world of raw light
so bright its camera blinded. Our story is a sea
of brave faces with grit teeth and shushed wings,

stalled hearts below glazed eyes. Our story is how
we did not shrivel though we were soaked,
we did not freeze in a cold almost beyond bearing.
Our story is we did not break and run—
no matter how close the lightning gouged.

SIDE RAILS

Dr. Stanislaw, did you know second-year nursing students
are only permitted to speak when asked a question,
attempt venipunctures if veins resemble sewer pipes,
and make rounds holding hands with head nurses?

Second-year blue uniforms have the bath down pat,
can figure doses, write care plans that instructors scar
with red slash marks. One Friday morning, I made rounds
with you and Miss Kitch on 6 East.

A family member asked you to please inform your silver-
headed patient, Miss Farley, that they could not possibly
care for her any longer, and a nursing home was the only answer.
We pulled the curtain; you lifted her blue-print gown,

exposing a sagging yeast-dough belly, now held fast
with black suture railroad crossings, a penrose drain—
everything healing well, and then, your hands gripped
her cool side rails, knuckles white:

Your family doesn't feel capable, the best place,
where you'll get good care, a nursing home
after you're discharged from here.
This was the dirty work I didn't know surgeons had to do.

I think damp rails will snap because your knuckles are blanched
so—your voice slices syllables—steady, scalpel thin.
You wish this molasses quiet were a rotten gallbladder,
a ruptured spleen, anything you could cut away.

Miss Farley weeps, soft, Baptist tears; for an eyelash moment
you hold her hand. On hairpin ceiling track, shushed curtain slides;
Miss Kitch sniffs, carries the chart, and I want to tell you—something,
standing under pure white and black clock hands weaving our gray lives

into honest shawls, I'd like to say, *Man, that was a shit deal,*
and you got class Doc, but I'm a second-year nursing student.
You are Chief of Surgery. No one asked me for an answer.
I'm just here to learn how 70% alcohol and ten Hail Marys
wipe silver rails clean again.

Father Damien

The son of a farmer, Father Damien was born in Belgium the winter of 1840. Following his brother's choice of vocations, he studied for the priesthood near Paris. Because he had typhus, Father Damien's brother was unable to fulfill his missionary service scheduled for the Hawaiian Islands, so Damien asked to go in his place. In the autumn of 1863, the seven-month voyage to Honolulu began, and two months after Damien's arrival, he was ordained.

In 1864 a leper colony was established on one of the poorest islands, Molokai. Soon after, a call went out through the church community for a priest to serve on Molokai. Father Damien quickly responded; he loaded livestock, supplies, and lepers and sailed the two hours to his new home. Upon his arrival, he found several hundred lepers, most of them dressed in rags, infected with sores, and living in huts. Through continuous efforts, Father Damien obtained lumber for better housing, installed a sewage system, and built schools, chapels, and orphanages. He served as engineer, carpenter, undertaker, nurse, and clergy. He stressed Christian values to the island inhabitants and converted many non-Catholics.

Living with and caring for the lepers, Father Damien noticed his own skin lesions early in 1877. In 1881 Princess Liliuokalani knighted Damien after her visit to the island. Though other priests visited the island from time to time, Ira

Father Damien, age 33, 1873. (Courtesy Library of Congress.)

Barnes Dutton, also known as Brother Joseph, was Father Damien's favorite assistant. As Father Damien's health waned, the Sisters of Charity sent a group of nuns to help Father Conrady and Father Moellers manage the settlement. Though his body grew gnarled and discolored, Father Damien's spirit remained calm. He died surrounded by his good works and followers April 15, 1889.

TO THE PLACE OF ORCHIDS

Father Damien, nurse to lepers, Molokai, 1864

The best orchid is small
and lives far away from the world.

What do I remember? Two men, dark as crows
in a field, cutting rows with their hoe.
Slow and sad, like giant tree frogs
who come out at dusk to climb skyward
the way prayer flies, unstoppable
toward heaven, knowing there's no hope.

Because of lost feet, one man had climbed
the other, who had no hands.
I felt my arms grow stone still, and my feet
fat against the grass. Brown hood and vows,
I sailed here, wanted to serve people
who would not look up.

Back and forth, row after row, peas, peas,
peas falling like rosary beads to feed
this village of fetid angels dressed in rags.
I stayed, lived in the middle of it, orange
blossoms, pure as a virgin's breast,
palm trees, perfect in the wind.

The sea was behind me, and I changed
years of bandages glistening with sap,
taken down every day like wires from their
limbs, sweet bodies ripening, rotting,
like pieces of fruit in a bowl, and me,
trembling under God's white, white clouds.

Some days, I wanted to scream,
Where is the sacred table and bread?
No Bible verse rose like bird song to help.
Caskets waved like lilies in my dreams.
No way to resist the Savior's shackles
to our ankles, our hearts.

I stood under the moon, doing my work,
told them to think orchids, nothing
but orchids, what we were, blooming
in this island's terrible sunset,
where we died, coming closer.

Rose Hawthorne Lathrop
(Mother Alphonsa)

$\mathcal{B}$orn in 1851 to a family that revered the arts, Rose Hawthorne Lathrop lived in London, Florence, Rome, Boston, and New York as a child. Her father was the famous novelist Nathaniel Hawthorne, and her mother, Sophie Peabody, was a painter and sculptor. Rose attended Kensington Art School in England. She was the youngest child in her family; her letters reveal a childhood filled with toys and traveling, but few playmates. Losing her beloved father one day before her thirteenth birthday created a wound that never completely healed. After her father's death, the family moved to Germany where Rose met George Lathrop, a writer and artist.

At age twenty, Rose married Lathrop. When Rose and George converted to Catholicism in 1891, it was a surprise to family and society. The marriage wavered and was never on solid ground after their only child, Francie, died from diphtheria when he was only four. By 1896 Rose was separated from her husband and studying to be a nurse at the New York Cancer Center. Essays written by Rose during this time period describe the city's impoverished families: tiny rooms packed with dirty children, a single bed, cupboards with no food, and the sick lying on chairs pushed together. Rose had lived comfortably, privileged; she felt this hunger as if it were hers and pleaded for those in government to address the plight of the poor. At age forty-five, she went to the Lower East Side of New York to find a house for nursing poor incurable cancer patients.

Rose Hawthorne Lathrop (Mother Alphonsa), 1893. (Courtesy Dominican Sisters of Hawthorne, Rosary Hill Home, New York.)

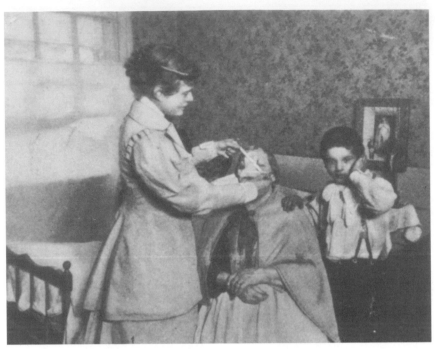

Rose Hawthorne Lathrop (Mother Alphonsa) caring for her patients, 1897. (Courtesy Dominican Sisters of Hawthorne, Rosary Hill Home, New York.)

Her life's course chosen, she used her writing skills to solicit funds from family friends and influential community leaders to support her hospice house. Though she wrote poems, memoirs, and short stories earlier in her life, the letters for her hospice work are the most impassioned. Her mission and its workload became well known and immense. Having heard of Rose and her works, in 1898 Alice Huber asked to be introduced to Rose. Soon after, Alice started working one afternoon a week with Rose. At first (Alice intended to stay only a few weeks) she felt called to "give her life to the work" and moved into the hospice. These two women shared a lifelong commitment to each other, their faith, and nursing incurable cancer patients. Eventually, they joined the Dominican order as tertiaries; Rose took the name of Sister M. Alphonsa, and Alice became Sister Mary Rose. As the hospice program developed, every challenge was addressed with prayer. If they needed land, Sister Alphonsa prayed for it and buried a medal on the site. She wrote more letters and begged for more money. Politeness was not an issue when they needed bandages, medicines, food, and beds. In 1900 the women were finally given the ceremony of profession and permitted to wear the black and white Dominican habits. The Servants of Relief had their own community and constitution.

In 1901 Mother Alphonsa purchased another property, which became known as Rosary Hill Home in Sherman Park. Here the patients were *incurable,* the beds *free,* and *no experimentation would take place.* To show the public and the patients how strongly they believed cancer was not contagious, no one wore gloves when caring for patients nor did they keep the patients' eating utensils separate from the staff's. The sisters did not beg for government money; they asked the general population to open their wallets and hearts to those who suffered poverty and disease. Mother Alphonsa explained their mission in essays and articles that appeared in popular magazines. The wealthy opened their wallets and gave generously. Sister Rose kept the books, and a pharmacist, Henry Reel, provided free medicine. Reel formed a six-hundred-member auxiliary for drugs; members contributed a dollar a year. A valued member of the Board of Trustees, he helped the sisters long after his retirement. This community was a wheel where all the connections were committed to caring for each other and their patients. A deep bond of affection between Sister Rose and Mother Alphonsa is evident in their correspondence and memoirs. In 1922 an article pleading for funds appeared in the *New York Times Magazine* because the sisters needed $200,000 for constructing a fireproof building. By 1926 they had collected $150,000, and the project was under way. Like countless nurses past and present, Mother Alphonsa went through her final day tending to patients and died in her sleep July 9, 1926. In 2003 Cardinal Egan of New York nominated Mother Alphonsa as a candidate for sainthood.

COVERING LILACS

Rose Hawthorne Lathrop, pioneer hospice nurse

As some women love flowers and border
their yards with lilacs instead of fences,
flank porches with roses, edge winding
brick paths with zinnias and hem gardens

with trillium, I live with those who bloom
lumps hard as sugar pears, clusters soft as grapes,
ulcers opening like tulips. I do not know why
a woman like me is called to tend people with cancer

or how I talked my friend Alice into helping.
She's a painter, an artist. Here we have snowless

mountains, each room coughs an angry fog.
Eyes ooze, like egg yolks, then dissolve.

Nothing for her canvas but ghost ponies
lathered and headed for a cliff. Some women
love dishes and fill their cabinets with china,
set the table with blue soup tureens.

Alice and I leave our door open, the way
a farmer does his barn. We curry each lame stallion,
unhalter the winded appaloosa, poultice
the mare's festered breast.

We do this with our bare hands,
we do not believe the word *contagious,*
do not believe in hiding shame with letters.
We cover our patients every day,

every night with cotton sheets
the way women spread tablecloths before the meal,
the way women cover lilacs before the frost.

Sister Elizabeth Kenny

The daughter of Australian homesteaders, Elizabeth Kenny was born in 1880. Described as a tomboy child and an adventuresome teen, she fractured a wrist after falling off her horse. It was when mending this injury that local physician Dr. Aeneas McDonnell showed her textbooks about muscles, and Elizabeth became determined to help her frail brother, William, strengthen his body. No doubt her success with his progress influenced her decision to become a nurse, and she chose to serve as an apprentice to a local nurse, Ms. Sutherland.

In 1911 rural families received Elizabeth's charity care, and this was the first year she encountered a child with polio. When she sent word to Dr. McDonnell, he told her, "Do your best." She applied warm wool blankets to spastic limbs and followed this with passive and active range-of-motion exercises. The child recovered without paralysis. Elizabeth successfully treated five more patients in one week.

Promoted from staff nurse to the rank of sister (first lieutenant) while serving as a World War I nurse, Sister Kenny was wounded in her knee by flying shrapnel. Over and over she witnessed trauma victims hemorrhaging to death. She invented a stretcher with wheels to prevent shock during transport of the severely injured from bush country, and the patent on the stretcher provided her income for the rest of her life. Wed only to her work, she was a pioneer single parent who adopted eight-year-old Mary Stewart in 1925.

Sister Elizabeth Kenny, 1943. Photo by Jack Delano. (Courtesy Library of Congress.)

Sister Kenny disagreed with the standard medical treatment of polio patients and began treating this population again in 1931. Labeled as a crackpot because her ideas of treatment were in opposition to those of the medical establishment, she was determined to get polio patients out of splints and on their feet. A trip to America in 1940 would convince the world finally that Sister Kenny's treatment was beneficial. In Minneapolis a large population of hospital polio patients were unsplinted and exercised with positive results. Physicians documented Sister Kenny's successful treatment in the *Journal of American Medical Association.* Countless polio victims were spared permanent paralysis because of this feisty nurse who refused to succumb to medical hierarchy.

ELSEWHERE SPARROWS: A NOTE TO SOME PHYSICIANS

Sister Elizabeth Kenny, Australian nurse who developed a new method for treating polio patients

I. She was no doctor.

Please understand women whose hearts are wagons,
how they must consider ambush or some outlaw
drunk and firing blindly
into their camp's small circle.

II. Parents begged.

Sister Kenny gathered children into her arms
like a bouquet, even when the bowed daisies
were knotted and lame, even when men told her
the roots were past coddling.

Look closely at women whose hands are plains,
how they teach themselves over and over to accept
whatever the ground gives, ignore aching backs
and limbs while doing the work of the fields.

III. She took no money.

There are women whose arms are oaks
giving graceful shade,

dropping acorns
for winter's squirrels.

IV. Her first clinic was a tent.

You have to study women whose pearls are sweat,
witness their yoke and branding, see how bread
is made with swallowed dust. There are women
whose lives are wells. They hang the tin cup
where it will catch the sun, welcome those who thirst.

V. She knew the body.

Sister Kenny was unpretty, but when she wrapped
the children's legs in warm wool blankets
and waited for spasms to cease, when she exercised tendons
stiff as broken fence rails, at last, the fawn was freed.

Still, some of you disbelieved her song
of water and blankets and hands.
There, in your eagle's kingdom,
does the eye have too much power?

Rita Maria Magdaleno

*B*orn in Augsburg, Germany, Rita Maria Magdaleno immigrated to the United States with her mother, a German war bride, in 1947. They traveled with green cards and alien registration numbers. Rita's earliest experiences—of living in Marcos de Niza, a South Phoenix housing project—are reflected in some of her narrative poems.

Currently Rita teaches poetry and autobiographical writing at the University of Arizona Extended University Writing Works Center. She has just returned from Germany, where she taught a class in contemporary Chicano literature at the University of Augsburg. Her newest poems appear in *Floricanto, Si! A Collection of Latina Poetry* (1998), and her book, *Marlene Dietrich, Rita Hayworth, and My Mother,* was published in 2003. She has been a writing fellow at the Millay Colony for the Arts in Steepletop, New York; the Ucross Center in Ucross, Wyoming; the Mary Anderson Center for the Arts in Mt. St. Francis, Indiana; and the Vermont Studio Center in Johnson, Vermont.

She graduated as a registered nurse from St. Joseph's Nursing School in Phoenix, Arizona, in 1968, where she was told she had to lose weight, "because nobody wants a fat nurse." She was weighed weekly and lost two dress sizes during training.

Although she has worked in diverse areas of medicine, she enjoys work in the healing arts. Through grant support from Rose Window for the Healing

Rita Maria Magdaleno, 1998. (Courtesy Rita Maria Magdaleno.)

Arts, she has led journal-writing workshops for women with breast cancer at the Arizona Cancer Center. Also, she facilitates "Writing for Renewal" workshops in Tucson, Arizona.

Teaching in school systems since 1991, Rita has served as poet-in-the-schools for the Arizona Commission on the Arts. Being on the Artist's Roster gives her rich opportunities to work with children and take literature into Arizona's rural communities. She lives in Tucson with her golden lab, Pachita, and has two children, Christopher and Regina, and two grandchildren, Hannah and Michael. She loves running rivers and hiking the Sonoran desert.

TEACHING WOMEN TO SPEAK

Rita Maria Magdaleno, nurse, creative writer

When I led the writing retreat
for women with breast cancer
I named it *Candlemas*—
moving toward the light,

because language is a lantern
able to lead women through darkness,
it allows pain to throw tantrums
in poetry's bed, cry itself to sleep
on the pillows of memoir.

I told the women to say
how it feels to pace chemo's porch,
offer burnt hair as sacrifice
and be the rose waiting
for the scissors' grin.

I watched them, women in bright
scarves, tired, but rising from ashes.
Their tears became stars
and the stars a string of rosary beads,
every day an answered prayer.

They were strong, but needed permission,
so I said it's okay, it's perfectly fine

to see cancer as a rabid dog.
They beat him blind with their pens,
with the only brooms they could still lift.

Part 2

I hear the Tsang-tsung road
Is rough and rugged, and hard to travel.
It is so steep that the mountains rise
In front of the rider's face,
And the clouds gather about the horse's head.

Li Po, "To His Friend Departing for Shuh"

Sandi Petek

$\mathcal{W}$ith more than twenty years of critical-care nurse experience, Sandi Petek is no stranger to a challenge. Drawn to nursing after high school graduation, she expected to get an education and join the Peace Corps. Sandi believes her mother was her greatest mentor and that her mother's love for traveling was contagious. Also, early in Sandi's career, she cared for a man who shared rich stories of living in Africa. A graduate of St. Alexis School of Nursing, this Cleveland, Ohio, native finds ways to dovetail her love for adventure and expertise as a nurse. In the past decade, she has been nationally selected for medical specialty teams who visited and cared for people in underdeveloped countries: Honduras (1990, 1993, and 1996), Guatemala (1990), and Viet Nam (1997).

On her first trip to Honduras, she served as the triage nurse, while the dental team cared for three hundred patients a day. The medical team learned to bathe in the river and shower under waterfalls. Wanting to learn how to make tortillas, Sandi rolled out at four o'clock one morning, drank "thick coffee with women in the village," and waited for them to start the dough. When she directed the beam of her flashlight to the basin where dishes were washed, she found out why her colleagues were getting gastrointestinal disorders: the dishwater had not been emptied for days.

Prior to leaving for any overseas mission, Sandi spends weeks collecting diapers, Bandaids, barrettes, baseball hats, toothbrushes and toothpaste, anything

Sandi Petek in Guatemala, 1991. (Courtesy Sandi Petek.)

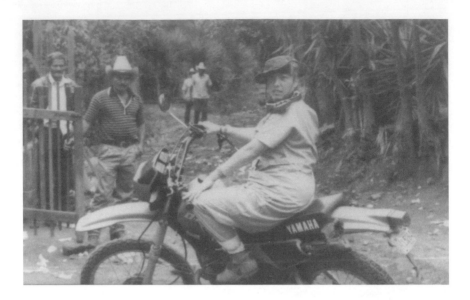

that promotes good will. She pays for most of her trips herself. While serving with an eye-care team in San Marcos, she offered patients a scapular of the Sacred Heart before cataracts were removed. All the patients were grateful and never flinched during their procedures, which amazed physicians and nurses. Counting surgeries, implants, prostheses, exams, and distributing donated eyeglasses, the eye team saw 8,500 patients in two weeks. The village women gave Sandi oranges and invited her to their houses for tea. In some areas the medical team stayed in farmhouses where forty people shared accommodations. If there was electricity, there might not be water. If there was water, it was cold and used for bathing only.

She has served as the camp nurse for children with cancer and cared for her father as he fought the same disease. "One night I was holding him with both arms, you know, trying to get him to the bathroom. I thought how we must look now, almost like dancers, the way it was when I was a little girl in my socks and would stand on his feet while he whirled me around the room teaching me the polka and fox trot." Her advice to new graduates is: "Use your common sense; follow your heart; look up what you don't know; that's why we have the books." This nursing dynamo has worked in hemodialysis units, dialysis units, emergency rooms, surgical intensive care, recovery rooms, flight nursing, and orthopedics. While she's not sure she'd become a nurse again, she is quick to admit, "It has been a fantastic journey."

VILLAGE

Sandi Petek, ER nurse, cleft lip/palate repair

Forty kilometers up the mountain
in Guatemala, you'll find it, a mining village
where the church is half voodoo, half crucifix,
and women in torn shawls bring their babies
to be blessed by the old priest. The challenge
is not the climb or being cut off from the world
by degrees or watching ox carts stumble on dirt roads
or knowing these brown faces are sons and daughters
of ten thousand towns you'll never see,
where poverty carves its name in rock and hardship's
the only language spoken. Being American,
you realize people change in before-and-after photos,
though it takes time for reconstruction
and for help to arrive when nature devastates.
The earth yawns and buildings collapse;
the Red Cross sends tents and hot soup.
Have you seen children born with notched lips
and palate spaces open through and through?
Such a force of nature happens
where there are no paved roads and health care's
a dream in a book no one can read. In the fullness
of summer, I traveled to such a place, a nurse,
a helper among a quiet group, working some magic
with my hands like a woman in her vegetable garden.
In my journal: *the houses have two rooms
(one for the Blessed Mother, one for the family),
the beans are as black as the kettles, parents ask,
"will my child look normal?" Every patient must pay,
a centavo, a peso, an orange, a goat. Bathing
in the river, I lost my soap. The stars are so close
I could pick them from the sky.* Our last day,
a farmer came: thirty years old, his face hiding
behind a scarf like a bandit. We lifted it
and saw the place God's soft hatchet had split
his smile. For six hours in a hallway chair
the plastic surgeons worked and worked,
only a local anesthetic. I held the man's hand,

wiped beads from his brow. He never moved.
He never moved. A local. Six hours. It's true.
It's all true. Yes. That's me in blue scrubs
with the village women by the door. I'm holding
the baby (she's two weeks old), the mother gave her
my name: *Sandi.*

Carlyann Markusic

*T*orn between a love for language and service to people, Carlyann Markusic has never turned her back on either. Born in Youngstown, Ohio, in 1945, she spent one year at Ohio State for nursing immediately after high school graduation. Then in 1966 she married and moved to northern Ohio, where her husband was employed.

Enrolled as the only married student in a diploma school (a hospital-affiliated nursing program), she felt "it [being a married student] was not viewed well. I did not live at the dorm. Once, I missed an exam because of a snowstorm, and one of my instructors told me 'housework and homework' don't mix." During her ten-week rotation at a rehab facility, she "had a rude awakening to real life" while caring for young men with multiple sclerosis and others paralyzed from diving or trauma. Some of her patients were angry because she was married. "They were young and now unable to perform sexually. They made lots of remarks about me going home for conjugal visits with my husband. I learned how to listen because these people were responding to the loss of their bodies."

Carlyann remembers the hardest thing in training was caring for psychiatric patients having electroshock therapy. "If it was their first time, they did all right, but the second or third time, they'd hold on to chairs, crying, begging me not to do it to them. I felt it was barbaric. Sometimes in nursing, you feel more like an accomplice than a caregiver." There were positive moments in her psych rotation. "On Wednesdays, we had dances for the patients, and everybody danced. Most nights, we'd play cards with them. They were very sharp at card games and never missed a beat. I was never afraid while working there."

An active member of the Ohio Nurses Association, Carlyann's nursing experience includes ten years in the emergency room, two years as clinical coordinator of the poison center, four years in the cardiovascular surgery recovery room, and nine years in a cardiovascular module. She also has three and a half years invested in an English degree at Youngstown State University. Impassioned with the thought that nurses need to be protected by fair labor rules, she has been involved with trying to organize nursing unions. Carlyann explains, "Nurses should not be switched around to cover unfamiliar clinical areas. Mandatory overtime is dangerous for nurses and patients. Nurses need the respect of their peers and other medical personnel. I'm discouraged with today's trend toward managed care and the replacement of professional registered nurses at the bedside with unlicensed assistive personnel." She has observed verbal and physical abuse of nurses over the years, and while it's reported properly, peer review favors physicians, not nurses. "Physicians mean money; nurses cost money. It's funny—I thought I would *never* answer *no* to becoming a nurse again, but at fifty-four years of age I feel that I am standing alone in what I think nursing should be and where it should be going."

STORY

Carlyann Markusic, former head nurse, emergency department

What's to tell? I worked ED, the head nurse
in a valley where my husband's steel mill folded,
our baby was four weeks old.

In a marriage, the reins pass back and forth,
two goldfish swimming in a bowl. The truth
is responsibility draws its own timetable—

episiotomy healed or not—and when the rent's due,
the landlord comes knocking. Yes, the black man
on our gurney had wrecked his Chevy. Joe, a local

policeman, kept asking, *Where's your license, man?*
I opened a dressing tray, some gauze,
poured peroxide, and told Joe,

It's there, on your clipboard Joe's eyes
went dark and hard, *Don't mess in my business,*
Joe snapped, he grabbed me from behind.

Have you ever seen it happen? How our lives tangle?
How anger stops negotiating and becomes a terrorist?
It's my name pin on the white uniform and Joe's gun

cold against my right temple,
a woman come back to work too soon,
an unarmed ship Joe wants to sink.

Joe yells, *I'll blow her away, I swear.* Two beds
over old Blinky Spell crawls on his knees,
whimpers, *Please don't hurt her, Mister.*

Blinky (who reeks of wine and stale smokes)
pleaded for my release, my life.
You know how they say, *Your whole life flashes?*

Don't believe it. I peed my pants, yeah, pure
yellow fear ran straight into my polished oxfords.
I wanted to cut a deal, wanted to wake up

the next day to dirty diapers and my husband's arms.
Code blue, room four, code blue. I said it,
and Marlene pushed a button with her knee.

Joe's captain came and some of his friends.
Yes, they knew Joe's wife had left
with some no-good trucker and his kids were sick

and his mother was nearly seventy, but they'd get
through it, help him, if he'd *put the gun down.*
Finally, he did. Blinky hugged my ankles and wept.

I'll bet if you're in prison and wet yourself
(say you're sick or just plain nervous)
the guards let you shower, get some dry clothes.

My supervisor, Mrs. Klemm, did just that:
Sorry, she said, *I can't let you go home;
there's no one to cover.*

but, go on down
to the doctor's lounge and shower,
grab a clean set of scrubs.

While I was in there, soap and water running hot
down thighs to the soft place where I still bled
from my son, I cried and cried and cried.

I could see his smooth pink face
how he was so small
and already able to wave his fists.

Sue Zenko

$\mathscr{A}$n honored graduate of Akron City Hospital's Idabelle Firestone School of Nursing, Sue Zenko admits her first career choice was law, but her parents encouraged her to become a nurse. "I'm the first person in my family to obtain a professional education. I applied for a nursing scholarship, and during the interview, the woman wondered why I was asking for money. 'Your father works at a steel mill, and he makes good money. Why are you asking for assistance?' I told her my father wasn't the one going to school, and I'd go to school with or without the scholarship. I got the scholarship." Sue remembers social assemblies in training "as a sort of finishing school; manners were taught; we had formal teas and wore gloves and hats. I never minded those gatherings."

As a student, Sue loved obstetrics, "though I got in trouble for searching through blankets until I found the very best for each newborn." Her pediatric rotation at Akron Children's Hospital was also very positive: "Children are uplifting, even if they are sick. The staff was very appreciative of students and often told us they couldn't get along without us." She was less enthusiastic about her three-month surgical rotation: "I really hated surgery. It seemed like an ego trip for the surgeons, and the rest of us were just handing stuff. Of course, I don't like equipment; even now, I don't have a lot of gadgets in my house, so maybe that was part of it."

Sue Zenko, 1997. (Author's collection.)

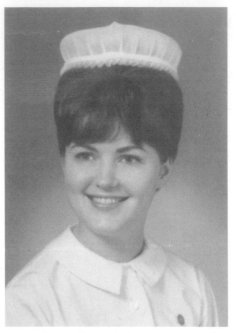

Sue Zenko, graduation, Akron City Hospital, 1966.

For her first year after graduation, Sue worked general duty at Akron City Hospital, married the next year and switched to office nursing. She was surprised the doctor asked her to resign when she was seven and a half months pregnant, "because he thought my pregnancy might be offensive to his patients." Like many mothers, she chose to be home with her three children when they were small. "I'm not part of the plastic-diaper generation. I sewed my baby diapers from flannel and ran a cake and cookie business out of my home. It was something I enjoyed, and I could do it on my own terms."

In 1985 Sue chose to reenter nursing, this time in a nursing home. Knowing she'd be challenged by changes at the newly built nursing facility, she discovered that the patients no longer seemed to be the focus. Administration drilled and stressed paperwork. She was constantly researching new medications, which were now packaged in single-dose units. "It was terrifying to go back to bedside nursing after being away so many years. We were oriented to the paperwork, but I needed to be updated on procedures and medications." Alzheimer's patients were not to be restrained, so it was a constant test of wills: "They would switch eyeglasses and shoes with each other; it was hard to keep track of them."

After one of the hardest months of her life, she resigned. While she never considered herself a "quitter," she found it impossible to be a part of what healthcare had become. "It wasn't nursing as I knew it, so I went to a Chinese restaurant, a place where I liked to eat, and asked them for a job. I was forty years old, and they were surprised I was interested in waitressing. They wanted me to be a hostess, but I refused. My job there lasted twelve years, and they were very flexible about my hours. I could work split shifts, go home and cook for my family, whatever I needed to do. I learned lots about Chinese food and people. The family members I worked with were very hard workers. In a way, it was like nursing. I was nourishing people, listening to people, but they were all healthy. I never hated going to work and made good money in tips."

Sue found herself very empathetic to people from different cultures trying to "make it in America." She reports, "I was nine years old before we had indoor plumbing, and my folks built a cement-block house." Sue is ambivalent about her decision to enter and leave nursing. She believes that "if patients were still the focus of nursing" she would still be a nurse, but "based on the horror stories [she] hear[s] from today's nurses, [she] couldn't do it."

This bright, active woman enjoys growing orchids, quilting, and collecting antiques.

WHAT HAS HAPPENED

Sue Zenko, 1965, Miss Student Nurse, Akron, Ohio

Miss Morley, I have left nursing
to waitress in a Chinese restaurant.

There are no old men peeing in wastebaskets
or young mothers bleeding from leukemia.

I earn more money in tips per week
than I did in wages at the nursing home.

I have learned to use chopsticks
and explain every dish on the menu.

Remember the little girl scalded in the tub
by her parents, and the broomstick

they somehow shoved up her rectum?
All these years I have tried and tried

to forget her crying in the night.
My mother is well; we don't dwell

on the three years I spent in Akron
to graduate first in my class.

What has happened to your blue hair
and white gloves?

Joanne Fowler

The mother of five children, Joanne Fowler was educated at the Allegheny Hospital School of Nursing in Pennsylvania. As far back as she can remember, her dream was to become a nurse. However, once she was a full-fledged student, she found coursework and instructors "so tough, very intimidating, and most of us [the students] were scared to death." She would come home and share her fears with her mother: "I know we could all do a better job, if we weren't so frightened." Like several others in her class, Joanne decided to quit one year shy of graduation. She challenged board exams for practical nursing and succeeded.

Raised in a rural community along with two brothers, she believes the first healer she observed was her mother. Her mother practiced common-sense care and home remedies like chicken soup. "We had a family doctor, but we didn't go to him very often." When her own children were young, one of her first jobs was with a family practitioner in a small town.

Later, while she was working in a nursing home, Joanne became enraged when one of her patients told her, "At night when I put the call light on, the nurse won't come and help me; she told me, 'If we don't get there in time, just go [urinate] in the bed.'" The patient was in a full body cast, had all of her mental faculties but no family to help her through the postoperative phase of her illness. Joanne resolved the problem and through her kindness became the patient's lifelong friend.

Joanne Fowler, 1998. (Author's collection.)

Joanne has also worked for the coroner's office, in emergency rooms, in pediatrics; and, since 1992, she's worked as a field nurse for the Cleveland Eye Bank. Her interest in organ donation surfaced in 1990 while she was working emergency. A young girl, an only child, was killed in a motor-vehicle accident. The girl's parents donated all her organs, and a New York doctor called the emergency room where Joanne worked immediately after the heart was successfully transplanted into a twelve-year-old girl. "I felt like I was witnessing a miracle," Joanne recalls.

Her job as a coroner's nurse was a six-month apprenticeship, or as nurses say, "See one, do one, teach one." Of course, if Joanne had a particularly challenging case, she did call on her mentor for assistance. Being the bearer of terrible news, she learned firsthand that the messenger is blamed for the tragedy. "Once a father picked up a chair and swung it around. I was ready to duck, but then he slammed it on the floor with all his might and started beating the wall. His son was killed in a car wreck. There's no easy way to tell people their loved ones are dead. It's not something you can rehearse."

After so many years, she still thinks the most difficult thing she's done in nursing was "giving my best friend an injection in training." Although her youngest son is a nurse, she "would not advise anyone to go into the field, because of all the pressure. I see what has happened to hospital nurses over the years. There's so much paperwork and not enough help. Hardly anyone has time to talk to me when I do an enucleation." For her, nursing was the right choice; "it's very natural for me to be caring and compassionate. I love helping others."

This vibrant woman is active in Bible study, sewing, square dancing, and reading.

ONE NURSE'S JOB: EYE RECOVERY ON A KINDERGARTNER

Joanne Fowler, nurse, eye bank

Nothing dares disturb this stillness.
A steel bed, no mattress, a five-year-old girl's
Orange dress, overhead, such brightness.
An awful light watches me lift the white swirl
Of sheet from her body. *I can do this,*
I tell myself. Six muscles hold each eye,
All must be cut, soft globes laid in a dish.
On paper, it is a notation, so why
Does this nurse shake? Forceps, scissors, gloves
Work the ball loose from its bony socket.

The brown ponytail shines, but I never loved
Her or held her smile inside my locket.
Tonight, a surgeon hugs his wife, laughs loud
Over barbecue. The eyeless make no sound
In his yard, and here, my tears keep trying
Not to be part of sterile procedure.

Rita Richards

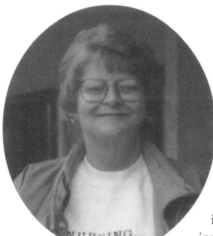

$\mathscr{A}$ registered candidate to become a chemical dependency counselor, Ohio native Rita Richards has been sober for nine years. Active in local recovery programs, she attends meetings and once a month leads group. The only female in a family of seven children, she vividly recalls her sixteen-year-old brother's battle with acute leukemia. Rita was fifteen at the time, and she watched his skin turn sallow; in six months, her brother was dead. Two years after this family tragedy, she enrolled in her high school's practical nursing program.

Students in this vocational program worked through the summer months doing clinicals at nursing homes and a local Catholic hospital. Rita remembers feeling very comfortable in the program because one of her aunts was a nun. The day she graduated from high school was her eighteenth birthday; she could practice nursing and had a full-time job waiting for her. Rita now acknowledges that at eighteen she was too young to shoulder the demanding responsibilities of nursing.

Her nursing career has included the following areas: med-surg units, cardiac, private duty, obstetrics, and geriatrics. Since 1994 Rita has been the day-turn charge nurse in a skilled nursing home, promoted to supervisor, and now handles Medicare issues in this facility. She feels a real cohesiveness with her staff, the physicians, and her patients. She recalls a challenging preemie, "Baby

Rita Richards, 1997. (Author's collection.)

Anna," whom she treated while working maternity in 1970, who weighed just over two pounds at birth. For three months Anna was the brightest light in the nursery; all the nurses fell in love with her. Anna thrived under their care and went home healthy.

Rita thinks that to facilitate community wellness nurses could band together and present public forums, free lecture series for new mothers and senior citizens, and question-answer hotlines. This softspoken mother of three does not plan on pursuing more nursing education because she believes each degree distances a nurse from the bedside. She enjoys crafts, baking, being a grandmother, and playing with her dogs, Missy and Bernie. When asked about her career choice, Rita doesn't hesitate to respond, "Yes, I'd become a nurse again. It [nursing] must have been God's plan. He made me pretty good at it. I belong."

TESTIMONY

Rita Richards, nurse, recovering alcoholic

The closet was loneliness.
I would crouch at the door and cry
as if I were in a trance, holding
my broken life in my hands.
For this type of wound there are no bandages.

Sometimes, your life cuts its wrists
to see if it can bleed, to see
if there's anything left of the soft center
of your being, the place layered with hurt.
It's dark, and you walk a spiral

chanting, *If there's anybody here, hold me,*
I'm scared; I'm so scared. Booze turned
me into an orphan who never said *no.*
How can a nurse be an addict? I asked myself.
Mother of three, I never drank or smoked

while pregnant, held a job and my babies.
My marriage was a broken cup tossed
into an alley. Habit of lies, rosary of tears,
a good Catholic girl raised by her grandparents
I tried to please. A nurse is supposed to be pure,

perfect. Though I didn't like the liquor's taste
I loved the way it made me feel—*alive*—a person
spinning without rules, a whirlwind.
Guilt was my brown sack and shame my bottle.
Being educated doesn't make you smart.

I had to drink to face her red eyes,
the trembling woman I met every morning
wearing my bathrobe, reeking of last night's bar.
I prayed for release, believed happiness was a bus
never bound for my street. The nightmare

swallowed me: days, weeks, months, years.
It mauled my children. Once, I fell into the tub,
and my six-year-old tried to pull me up.
A Mommy drowning in blackouts, a broken kite
unable to fly. In treatment, there's a chair

called *hot seat*. The group grilled me until
I gushed: milk puddles dot the kitchen, my kids
ate Cheerio suppers, fell asleep to TV, wild parties,
men with sour breath and dirty hands, it's a guess
who was driving the night we wrecked, but the pain

was real, it was raw, and finally, I knew
if something didn't change, I'd die.
I couldn't survive in a neighborhood
where fear ran in packs and ate
out of garbage cans at twilight.

So, I had to leave and let it hurt.
In a clear voice, I can tell it now,
how I learned to stand, without an apology.

Pat Austin

One of twelve children, Patricia Austin grew up in a house where sharing was the key word. She believes children in large families learn to nurture and care for one another and take on different roles as the need arises. Immediately after high school, Pat was pursuing an education in x-ray technology. Having completed one year of study, she was involved in a serious motor-vehicle accident and had a long hospitalization, which forced her to withdraw from her studies for one year. When she returned to her education, she switched to nursing and graduated from Akron City Hospital's Idabelle Firestone School of Nursing.

Assisting in the delivery of a baby girl led to her meeting the man she would marry. Family members waited for news of the birth, and Pat's future husband, Tom, was the baby's uncle. Pat remembers the delivery as "her best day in nursing." She also speaks highly of her obstetric instructor, Mrs. Wilson, "who enjoyed nursing so much and was such a fine teacher, she made us all love it." As a med-surg nurse for four years, she witnessed the beginning of many changes in hospital nursing. There were fewer hands to carry the workload. After having her children, she worked part-time, and she remembers, "I'd get all fretted up on the days I had to work because I knew there was so much to do and I was afraid of making an error. I'd have to live with that."

It's difficult to name one moment that makes a career turn a corner, but

Pat Austin, 1997. (Author's collection.)

caring for an eight-year-old boy who died from leukemia had a lasting effect on Pat. "I had spent time with this young man, reading and playing games; he had a tremendous insight and courage." She realized how closeness to patients translates to suffering for nurses. Mindful that she should protect herself, she started considering other nursing specialties. Her neighbor worked at a large facility for mentally retarded and developmentally delayed clients "who always need nurses." Pat applied, was hired and has cared for this population for sixteen years. "It's a similar scenario with this population. They have one problem after another. The children born with Down's syndrome end up with Alzheimer's when they are forty or fifty years old. Parents want to dictate the care of their children, and often the administrators give in." The trend today is for mentally challenged children to stay with their families as long as possible. Presently, the youngest resident in Pat's workplace is eight years old. "We do a lot of teaching; we teach clients to say the names of their pills, to take their pills, to know why they take their pills and how to pack their pills." Every relationship starts with trust, and that takes time with any child or adult. Activities of daily living are constantly being taught to clients. Pat shares: "We want everyone to function at their highest possible level and reward appropriate behaviors."

When asked to comment on the nursing profession today, she says "Nurses should earn more [money] than what they have in the past because what a nurse gives to an ill patient is invaluable." She also regrets medicine's current revolving-door patient care. "I would want to see more hands-on nurses, and we have gotten away from that kind of nursing care. When you leave the hospital right away, you have to hope that you have family and friends to help care for you. I realize cost must be considered, but the present method may cost us a lot more in human life." She recalls her mother and aunt telling their nurse stories when she was a youngster; some were funny and some serious. Pat admits some of those stories might have influenced her career choice, though she says she would "probably not become a nurse again, though I'm not sure what I'd do without nursing."

A BOAT THEY FLOAT IN

Pat Austin, nurse, MRDD facility

Outside each classroom: *children's wheelchairs*
(say it—say it again and again). What wounds
the heart fights the tongue. Small black chariots
sit below bulletin boards blooming

wild pastel flowers on manila papers.
The strangeness of all artists, watch the brown
girl, how she chews her arm like a chocolate bar
or the willowy jazz drummer's bent grin,

frothy from years of wool carpet gigs.
Song of Solomon, Song of Soft Moans.
Where are the mothers to claim this son?
Imagine having pain and no word for it

(it happens all the time), but here the sign
for *hurt* is index fingers lined up touching.
The retarded are more disposed to happiness—
it's a boat they float in. Still, we coax

them into the water, want them to relax.
They learn the weight of competition
and the dazzle of medals. Up close,
the princess is not always pretty, easier

to see her ruffled dress sway back and forth
from the ceiling's hammock, easier to say,
She's pricked her finger, under a spell,
the eggnog stuff dripping in her tube's

a hunk of melted star, medicine to wake her
from an awful dream. If you believe in music
and mountain sunsets, then believe this: children
return to the world dressed as butterflies.

There's soil piled in the greenhouse, and spastic
hands press seedlings into cups. Moon-faced farmers
do the miraculous: they smile in a rainless valley.
Magicians, they wave hoses like wands.

Inside the workshop, residents put gray pipes
into boxes, put gray pipes into boxes. Show me
one life that doesn't fill with repetition.
At this complex, no planes take off.

Toys must be labeled: DOLLHOUSE, TRUCK, DISHES.
What does it mean to wash your hands and get a hug,
count your days by seizures, wear your ponytails
under a red helmet, this life of little rest?

Consider Michelangelo straining on his scaffold,
the veined protest of aching arms, how hard
it is to paint angels, angels, and Mary's goodness,
her baby always pink, flawless.

Elfriede Anton

*B*orn in Vienna, Austria, the winter of 1916, Elfriede Anton dreamed of becoming an architect. Once accepted into a school for this course of study, she spent the first month sweeping floors and applying stamps to envelopes. Disheartened, she told her parents, "I quit." When her father suggested nursing as an alternative career, she agreed to try it. Elfriede remembers the students wore dark stockings and blue veils. She worked with disturbed children, and at bedtime every child received a heaping spoon of Phenobarbital.

Her religious roots are both Jewish and Catholic: her grandfather was the son of a rabbi, her grandmother was Catholic. From this union, six girls were born. Three of the girls were raised Jewish, and three were raised Catholic. Elfriede's unmarried aunt served as the family nanny while her mother worked in business. The family's upper-middle-class status could not shield them from the German secret-service patrol; Elfriede's physician uncle was shot. She recalls how old people, lawyers, and doctors were forced to scrub streets with rags at gunpoint. "Friends just disappeared; it was a very bad time." Her father was taken prisoner in Dachau, and after weeks of negotiations, young Elfriede secured his release. "I still don't know how I did it; he was a blue-eyed Jew."

Helped by Quakers, Elfriede and her parents escaped their beloved Austria, bound for different countries; her parents went to America, and she went to

Elfriede Anton, 1997. (Author's collection.)

Elfriede Anton's nursing diploma, 1936. (Courtesy Elfriede Anton.)

England. Once in America, Elfriede's parents tried unsuccessfully to get her brother, Kurt, out of Austria. In England, Elfriede hoped to reconnect with her fiancé and settled down to a job as a nanny. At three o'clock in the morning, Elfriede arrived to her new job by train. A man delivering newspapers offered her a ride. She had an address, and one hour later she reached her destination. In darkness she sat on her suitcase and waited for her new family to wake. In the beginning, she was unable to work as a nurse in England, though she dressed like one when caring for her employer's children. Later, she was a seamstress in a garment factory, and when she told stories of occupied Austria, people refused to believe her. She was eventually reunited with her Austrian fiancé and married. When he joined the English army, both of their titles were upgraded to "friendly alien." Thus labeled, Elfriede was allowed to work as a midwife in the remote hills of England.

In 1951 Elfriede, her husband, and two children arrived in America, where her mother told her, "Everyone works." She went to work at Saint Francis Hospital in Peoria, Illinois, as an obstetrical nurse. Well-liked by the physicians, she received a scholarship and went back to college, and in three and a half years she earned a dual degree in sociology and German. When she thinks about Austria, she remembers the lovely fountains her family designed and the bags of broken pastries a child could buy for a dime. The mother of three children, Elfriede feels "we must forgive, but never forget." She keeps her mind and body sharp by swimming twice a week, reading, traveling, and serving her church community.

UNDERGROUND: A NOTE TO MY BROTHER, KURT

Elfriede Anton, retired obstetric nurse

How not to forget our Vienna, 1941,
the waltz put aside for a war, the castles quiet,
so many stiff dancers and cold menorahs.
How to forgive the neighbor man, a spider waiting,
watching Aunt Katrina sneak a boy's shirts from the clothesline,
cuddle round breads inside her coat.
From her cellar the SS dragged you, stomped your eyeglasses.
Why didn't you leave with Leo? He made it to Israel.
The Jews in America refused Papa a loan to get you here.
How to go on loving Rilke, knowing your story
was buried in the camps.
Remember how Mama's flowers hugged each other
at the weekend house? How Papa told us to always share
our strawberries at school? I have children, grandchildren.
An old lady of fifty, I returned to college. Sometimes,
I saw you on the campus, your arm tight around a girl,
your blue eyes whistling.

Theresa Marcotte Kokrak

A native of North Bay, Ontario, Canada, Theresa Marcotte Kokrak is accustomed to adverse conditions. She recalls leaving for hospital duty in blizzards, in seventy-below wind-chill weather, as part of her life's landscape. As a youngster Theresa severely burned her foot with boiling water. Her mother served as doctor and nurse for the injury, and the foot healed without incident. Although North Bay has a high population, the people are spread out over a large area, and folks don't run to the hospital over every drop of blood.

In high school Theresa thought about becoming a teacher or a nun, which would mean going away to college. Economics were a big part of the family equation, so she decided to stay in her hometown and become a nurse. "My sister was a nurse, so I became a nurse," she says. Earning a scholarship in grade thirteen helped defray expenses for her nursing education at Canadore College of Applied Arts and Technology in North Bay. Maintaining an admirable grade point average, Theresa was granted a scholarship every year in training.

Early in Theresa's career, she took a job at a large psychiatric hospital in a rural setting where all the patients were below age thirty-three. Until she worked closely with this population, she wondered if psychiatric patients might just be "faking it." How could people who looked "so normal" be "so sick"? Once while making her nightly rounds Theresa discovered that a patient had deliberately set her bed on fire: "The flames were nearly to the ceiling, so I just threw a

Theresa Marcotte Kokrak, 1998. (Author's collection.)

blanket over them, doused the mattress with water, and smothered the fire before it spread." She burned her hands in the process and was reprimanded for not calling the fire department and following hospital procedure. Feeling her positive energy waning, she decided to change jobs.

As an obstetrical nurse, Theresa worked closely with midwives and physicians, gaining knowledge about high-risk mothers and infants. Physicians would place their hands over Theresa's and teach her how to palpate a term uterus. "See, here's the head, and if the baby is transverse, we're in trouble. If you ever think something is wrong with one of my patients, I want you to call me." One very memorable delivery with which Theresa assisted was a blind, bilateral amputee. "The husband was so supportive and the mother (who was a brittle diabetic) was so happy. It was a blessing to be in the room with them," she says.

When she moved to the United States, Theresa experienced culture shock. Not only were the drugs different, the physician-nurse relationship was very hierarchical. She felt the nurses were verbally abused and wondered why such behavior was acceptable. She reports, "In Canada, the medical community functions more like peers."

Holding on to her integrity, she's proven to be an asset in her communities on both sides of the border, serving in the following areas: obstetrics, psychiatric units, intensive care, emergency room, and urgent care. This mother of two sons feels "the privilege of being a mother and a nurse is a gift from above."

TO SAVE WHAT WE MOST LOVE

Theresa Marcotte Kokrak, critical-care nurse

Building other men's dreams
in morning's half light,
Dad worked construction.

His right arm dangled,
a sickly rope he'd pocket hide
after the windy fall.

For dinner, I went to wake him;
he was lavender's groom,
pale and wooden on the bed.

I screamed
and placed my mouth to his,
a bear tore through my chest,

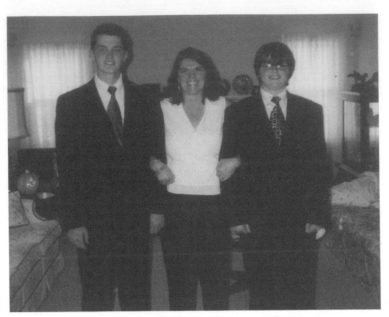

Jason, Theresa, and Matt Kokrak. (Courtesy Theresa Kokrak.)

my lips, my breath, his daughter's breath.
I laced my hands and pressed his ribs
down and down and down

squeezed his clotted heart,
one spoon had fed us all,
a red grenade, exploded.

Medics came and called him *dead*.
They said, *The bed's too soft,*
best to drag them to the floor.

I didn't say, *He was a mountain*
in a flannel shirt. No. I folded
the room's smallness, a maple stand

holding its sky blue lamp
and my parents, newly married,
smiling inside the oval frame.

Terri Swearingen

*D*edication and determination are both accurate words to describe Terri Swearingen's approach to community problems. Since she graduated in 1978 from the Ohio Valley Hospital School of Nursing, Terri's medical knowledge has been a helpful tool for local and national environmental agencies. Since 1990, she has worked tirelessly to monitor a toxic-waste incinerator built near her hometown of Chester, West Virginia. "When the talk started about building an incinerator in East Liverpool, I couldn't believe it. We live right on the Ohio River, and jobs are scarce. Sometimes, people equate jobs with smokestacks. The incinerator managers promised employment and free electricity. The proposed site was so close to our school. It seemed like we had been chosen as a *sacrifice zone*. I just had to do something."

Along with other concerned citizens, Terri researched emissions standards, local cancer rates, national experts in toxic waste, and ways to halt building the incinerator, a modern-day monster threatening families in three states. "There were public hearings, but they wanted to limit citizens to five minutes. We wanted experts to testify, so we relinquished our time to the experts. One of our witnesses testified for more than two hours. He said the dioxin and mercury levels would be too high with the proposed burners. When the test burns were done in 1993, his prediction was correct: dioxin and mercury levels were too high. Another system had to be added to the incinerator to counteract these unacceptable levels."

Terri Swearingen, 1995. (Courtesy Terri Swearingen.)

Physicians and environmentalists, grandparents and labor leaders, spoke publicly against the incinerator. "We went to the Ohio Environmental Protection Office in Columbus and *pink-slipped the workers* [symbolically fired them] because they weren't doing their jobs. They weren't protecting our community." Later, Martin Sheen, actor and member of Greenpeace, met with Terri to gather more information about the problems facing her community. In one peaceful demonstration, more than a thousand people from West Virginia, Ohio, and Pennsylvania joined in the Hands across the River protest. "In 1992, we had a week of events where every day a different community group lined up in front of the incinerator gates to protest: grandparents in rocking chairs, parents, labor leaders, teachers, medical professionals (they used cast material to bandage the gates shut), and small business organizations. All of us were arrested. We constantly wrote letters to the White House asking for help. The response was like a form letter, so we decided to go to the president's house."

Having grown up by the river, Terri realizes the fragility of a flood plain and speaks nationally and locally about her concerns regarding the consequences of an "accident" at any incinerator. Her goal is to educate people about the real threat of toxic waste to existing and future generations. A former office nurse, Terri has left nursing to focus on the environment: "I'm just an ordinary person, but I believe in divine intervention." Two of her many awards are the 1993 Ohioan of the Year and the 1997 Goldman Prize for North America, the latter of which is the highest environmental award given in North America. She now serves on the board of Greenpeace.

This wife and mother states, "No child in America should have to go to school eleven hundred feet from a toxic waste incinerator, and no president should allow it."

THE EVOLUTION OF LIGHT: EAST LIVERPOOL, OHIO, SITE OF THE WTI INCINERATOR

Terri Swearingen, nurse, environmental activist

Do you see any tents along this river?
We are not nomads. A fixed community
cannot ignore garbage crematories.

I am a housewife, a nurse, a mother.
To protect my family, I've been to jail,
pink-slipped the EPA, written the president

over and over. He wouldn't come here,
so we went to his house, sat in the Grand
Ballroom singing, praying. Secret Service

agents have a special way of bending wrists;
they can snap them if they want. The D.C. jails
were awful: vomit on the toilets, roaches,

a young black girl hung herself with her bra.
I grew up here, was a cheerleader, my daughter's
fifteen. Poisoned land doesn't come clean.

What's flushed into the sky funnels back
to our bodies, lands like a seed in the pancreas,
filters down to our lungs. How long until

we cough the red petal or find the almond
while showering? Whose sister will bear
the first son without an arm? Let it be entered

into the records even the unemployed understand
dioxin and mercury are nothing like moldy lettuce
or rotting grapes. I am a nurse, a mother, a housewife.

We live on a hundred-year flood plain, still
the EPA let this incinerator be built 1100 feet
from our school. Maybe one of our kids is another

Madame Curie or Mozart. Sleep. I don't get a lot
of sleep. Letters. Rallies. Handcuffs. Policemen
watching X-rated movies. Rain comes to our valley

when it must, not knowing clouds are boils
filled with pus. So far, fifteen days in jail
(one was Christmas Eve). I grew up here—

this is America, 1997. We are making buttons,
banners, holding hands across the bridge,
planning to go over the fence.

Helen Albert

𝒯he granddaughter of a slave, Helen Albert was born the spring of 1921 in Argo, Alabama. Her grandmother was one of three black children purchased on a North Carolina auction block by a young white couple who were abolitionists. The couple told the children "if you come to Alabama, help us work our farm, stay with us through old age and death, the hundred acres we now own will be deeded to you." That is exactly what happened, and for three generations, the farm has remained in the family.

Helen is no stranger to tragedy: her father died when she was an infant, and her family cabin burned down when she was three. After this, with her mother and brothers and sisters, Helen moved in with other family members on the farm. "Wherever we lived, that was home. I was treated like a daughter in any house I lived. It was just that way." The nearest hospital was thirty miles away, and many people didn't even own a mule. Helen's mother was a midwife, often called out in the middle of the night. "We were never allowed to go with her; it was a sacred time for her and the new mother."

Having grown up on a farm, Helen remembers harvest time and canning three hundred to four hundred jars of vegetables, fruits, and meats. The extended family stored them all in a ground shelter known as a storm pit. They heaped sweet potatoes in mounds "like an igloo with straw around them, so they wouldn't freeze. When you slow bake sweet potatoes in raked ashes and

Helen Albert, 1997. (Author's collection.)

put fresh butter on them—nothing tastes better." Her mother cooked biscuits for breakfast and cornbread for supper. The iceman came twice a week. And her mother made lye soap from hog grease. "We had a huge black pot to boil our clothes in until they were white. There wasn't any washing machines."

After graduating from high school, Helen went to work for Dr. and Mrs. W. B. Martin. They knew how she longed to become a nurse and encouraged her dreams. Once admitted to Norwood Hospital School of Nursing, Helen lived with the other black nursing students on the first floor of the dormitory. The black patients stayed on the first floor of the hospital. There were no black physicians in her hospital, but all the students were "treated well by the hospital staff." Helen's mother taught her "to stand up for right and do your best to be outstanding."

Helen's life mirrors those words. In 1944, she and her husband moved to Ohio. Here he would get a job in a steel mill and she would become "the first black registered nurse hired in Warren, Ohio." The mother of two sons, Helen worked for fourteen years at St. Joseph's Riverside Hospital, where she was continuously promoted until she became the nursing supervisor of the entire facility for three years. This softspoken woman credits her life's work of building—first a nursing home, then a facility for the mentally retarded, and later a community center in Alabama—and serving as a role model of "loving, sharing and caring" for other women. "As many white people as black use the community center," Helen states. "And if we can't get along together here on earth, God won't want us in heaven." A person of strong faith, Helen has many awards, including Warren's Woman of the Year, 1965; Outstanding Community Service from Warren Urban League, 1972; Honorary Mayor of the City of Warren, 1974; one of the Outstanding Women of the World, 1975; Community Leaders and Noteworthy Americans Award, 1975–1976; listed in 1976 Bicentennial Edition of Notable Americans of the Bicentennial Era; International Who's Who of Women, 1979; Who's Who of American Women, 1979–1980; Susan B. Anthony Award, 1980 (by Shriners and Imperial Court Daughters of Isis); and Warren Urban League Award for Outstanding Community Services, 1980.

JUBA

Helen Albert, retired nursing supervisor

Not the gray truck bound for the cotton fields
or the thirty-mile mornings dark riding cold,
not the sweet biscuit smell twisted in Mama's hair
or the dull flowered dresses stretched

to cover bare legs. Closer and closer,
our coats were whispers, straw hats frayed,
hands literate in the energy of motion.

Not the oval slowness of filling hundred-pound
sacks or the backs' silence wanting to walk away,
not the soft hymns singing themselves across
hired rows of squatters. No. Not the mechanics
of stops and pauses, day labor without shade,
but the clean taste of water from our own jugs,
the sense of purpose given to those who work.

Not the parlor chairs or starched linens
or cherry staircase of Dr. Martin's, not waiting
on his porch for my three dollars. No. The day
he went to Norwood Hospital on my behalf,
the Monday I was one of eight black women accepted
for nurse's training. Yes. That afternoon, and the Sunday
Mama's best friend, Hannah, pulled white sheets

From her bed to sew my uniforms. The coal miners'
paychecks handed over by my uncle and brother
to buy my nursing shoes so I might have the power
to lift the raw material which was my life.
I'm seventy-six years old, and at this distance
the pieces come together, one thing embraces another,
clover and fences and creeping grass, suppers of salt pork

And warm beans over cornbread, wooden ironing boards
holding the dead until a box was built. Me, learning
hard lessons of science and logic, finding the narrow strip
of light where God lets everything grow,
how I graduated first in my class at Norwood,
a black woman in Alabama in 1943,
at the southern rim of Appalachia,

Not sailing as far as the Cape of Hope,
but a place where the growing season can be long,
and girl, you must be glad for rain, straw layered
around the community of jars in the storm pit,
any old cow still able to give milk.

Esther Baker

A southern Ohio farm girl born in 1920, Esther Baker learned the importance of helping others by observing the behavior of her family and folks in her surrounding community. Her father's 110-acre farm provided crops, meat, and plenty of beauty for Esther and her four siblings. However, the one thing her family, like most farm families, was usually short on was cash. Knowing her dream was to become a nurse, her father secured a special bank loan to pay for her education at White Cross Hospital School of Nursing in Columbus, Ohio, and Esther paid him back after training.

Esther clearly remembers the black stockings and shoes worn by students during their probation, and how transformed she felt when she received her white cap in the hospital chapel ceremony. She does recall some trying times during her student experiences. Once, in the operating room, a surgeon threw a pair of hemostats across the room and shouted, "Where'd you get those things? They're no good!" Then he asked, "Little girl, where are you from?"

She gulped and answered, "La Rue, Ohio."

"Do you know Lester Smith?"

"Yes."

"Well, I bought my dogs from him." After that, the surgeon and Esther got along just fine.

While working a surgical floor, Esther became attracted to one of her patients.

Esther Baker, 1997. (Author's collection.)

After his release, they dated, fell in love, and were married. When she and her husband moved to Newton Falls, Ohio, she worked as a private-duty nurse for four dollars a day. Many nurses did not want to care for craniotomy patients because the outcome was bleak, but Esther welcomed the challenge. She would assist in the operating room and provide care for them in their postoperative days. After her son was born, Esther accepted a position as an occupational health nurse in town, but she quit after six months because nothing seemed more important than caring for her baby.

A survivor of colon cancer, Esther has only praise for the male nurses who cared for her after her surgery. "They were compassionate and very caring." While working obstetrics in the 1940s and 1950s, she remembers the patients "were wild from scopolamine; they would stand up in the beds and beat on the walls; we had to take care of them one-on-one, and it was very scary." Fathers were not allowed in the delivery rooms.

There is no doubt in Esther's mind that she would become a nurse again: "It gave me great satisfaction to help other people—that was my goal." Over the years, many patients thanked her for caring so deeply; occasionally she received cards or short letters. This note was received by Esther Baker from one of her patients.

May 27, 1941
Dear Esther:

You should see our little Danny now. He weighs over 8 pounds and is 21 inches high. Considering his tinyness when born don't you think he's made a good gain the first month. He is asleep now but will wake him for his bath as soon as I finish writing. Sunday we took him to his Grandpa B for his first visit. He was a very good boy and is most of the time. He sleeps well at night and we are thankful of that.

I was just out walking around in our yard. My, how pretty the flowers are! I wish you could see them too, for I know that you like flowers. Pyrethrum, Oriental poppies, aquilegia, Digitalis, Forget-me-nots, Delphinium, and Sweet Rockets are all in full bloom. My Canterbury Bells are almost out too. Last but not least I have around 60 different colors of iris in bloom now. I am surely glad that I could come home when I did and see all the lovely flowers. It made me appreciate them all the more.

I want to thank you again for your services rendered me while I was at Green Cross. If all nurses were like you it would surely be a swell place to go. We want you both to come see us as we enjoy having our friends come to visit us. You just write and tell me when you can come so we will be sure to be at home. I do hope that your work does not get too hard and that you have many pleasurable times this summer.

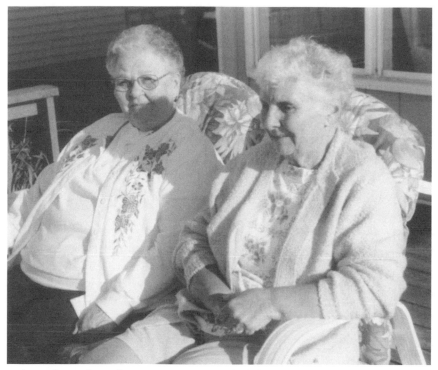

Esther Baker and Josephine Montgomery. (Author's collection.)

We have had over 100 different people (young and old) to call at our home to see our little Danny. He has a card table stacked three feet high of presents and they are nearly all different things. Almost everything you can think of. His Aunt Verlene has taken out life insurance for him and is going to keep it paid up. I don't even have life insurance. Do you? Thanks again and hope to see you sometime soon.

Your friend in room 210,

Mrs. B.

LETTER TO JOSEPHINE, 1996

Esther Baker, retired occupational health nurse

Dear Jo: Today I read an article about some explorers who died trying to climb Mt. Everest. An unexpected snowstorm. Two were women. They left base camp thumbs up, smiling beneath a rainbow twirl of prayer flags. The Sherpa believe when the wind blows the cloth, prayers rise to heaven. They say when a person's freezing the discomfort's a sort of numbing; she dreams, then goes to sleep. As nurses, we both know there are worse ways to go. Did you know the first expedition reached the summit in 1953? The same year I stayed with you through the delivery. Remember our houses on Orchard and Bane? All the steps from the cellars to the kids' rooms upstairs? How I'd like to hurry over one more time and help you gather the sheets before it rains. That year, February made snow mattresses for every garage. Sometimes, when it's winter and dark, I go back to the black phone ringing and your husband, Tom, saying, *Jo's water just broke. Can you come, Esther?* I take the steps two at a time in my flannel nightie, brush my bangs, and dress. In the back seat, you shiver, and your hair's damp sable brown. We fix a towel under your coat. With a blanket my arms circle you, and we half rock, hold each other while your body releases pain's song like shavings beneath a lathe. Inside you, a great pole pushes, and there's no walling it off. At the hospital, they send Tom way down the hall with other men who smoke Lucky Strikes, sip bitter coffee, and pretend to read. What can we tell them about *this* anyway? How a woman crawls into it for so many hours? How her breathing becomes salve for the seismic waves of her uterus? This is women's work, the margin of death and life, the dance of sisters beside a cliff, holding hands until the pushing and panting of one person becomes two, and you see the top of the world—a little daughter, a pink moonflower, so beautiful when you hold her we weep with joy. It's been too long between letters and walks with you at the lake's cabin, old friend. Take care, Esther.

Part 3

❧

Each cell has a life.

ANNE SEXTON
"IN CELEBRATION OF MY UTERUS"

A peasant's house, the kitchen table, candlelight
All night the men work at her body.
Stiff as a plank, she is hard to undress.
Villagers claim a priest fathered her child.
Shame drove her to the river; she rose
After three days, a salmon with silky hair,
Her baby's fists still clenched inside.
She feels, somehow, softer when the knife opens
The white cage of her breast bone
And warmer when they spread her wide.
Their hands are a meat-cutter's: bloody and crude
They drink wine to make it easier
And try not to see her hair spilling
Like ink almost to the chair.
Until dawn they hack and cut and lift.
They place the heart and fetus
In separate sacks, smaller than pillowcases
But clean, very clean. Because she
Was not a criminal, what they've done
Is against the law, but Leonardo's an artist.
They drag the woman to their cart, dump her
Back into the hole. Her arms flop and twist
And snap under her hips.
She cannot cover this huge emptiness.
They shovel the earth upon her, dirt,
Dirt, dirt, and cold, like brown pearls.
Now Leonardo draws her heart's chambers,
Each vessel's breathless chimney,
And her baby hugging his bent knees.
Art takes everything, digs for secrets,
Ravages the queen's tomb to seize her gems.
It leaves nothing in the unlit house,
But silence and stains upon the floor.

MISCARRIAGE: THE NURSE SPEAKS TO THE BABY

We are going back to the dirty utility room,
you floating like a ballerina in a jar, and me,
wondering how you found an open space in the woods.
Little gardenia, you have split your mother's heart.

To make a baby for this world, women spin
a film of scarlet cobwebs inside themselves;
they ask a blessing, to become a gourd,
a field where grain is grown.

You are the dancer whose rhythm is not metrical,
and I name you abandoned flute.
You are the tiny globe of two worlds, and I hold you,
a pale candle too wet to light.

You are the journey unwilling to go forth,
watercolors touching the sky, spices
from a faraway land, daughter of silk and air and dawn,
vine of warm ground born to suffer loss.

Maude Callen

*O*ne of thirteen sisters and orphaned by age six, Maude Callen was born in Quincy, Florida, in 1898. Reared in the home of her physician uncle, Dr. William J. Gunn of Tallahassee, she graduated in 1922 from Florida A&M University and later from the Georgia Infirmary in Savannah. She married William D. Callen in 1921. Called to be a missionary nurse, she moved with her husband to Berkeley County, South Carolina, in 1923 for a temporary position, which would last a lifetime. Miles from any hospital, the Callens built a house and eventually added two rooms to serve the community as a clinic. Maude trained to be a nurse-midwife at the Tuskegee Institute in Alabama and became an asset to the local physician.

Life in her new county was hard; at the edge of Hell Hole Swamp in Pineville houses were still lit by oil lamps, not electricity. Not having power lines meant no telephones, and people went to town by wagon or buggy. Here, over the years, Maude taught many women to be midwives. Each session opened and closed with a hymn, and she conducted monthly refresher classes.

Maude made her rounds in a four-hundred-mile area, and she frequently had to park her car and walk through mud, woods, and creeks to reach her patients. By 1936 she held the position of public health nurse in the Berkeley County Health Department, making her responsible for the children in nine schools. Her duties included vaccinations, examinations, and keeping records

Maude Callen, 1983. (Courtesy Wade Spees, Charleston Post and Courier.)

on the children's eyes and teeth. It is estimated she delivered between six hundred and eight hundred babies in her sixty-two years of practice. In 1951 *Life* magazine's W. Eugene Smith's poignant story about her community work prompted readers to donate enough money to build the Maude E. Callen Clinic in Pineville, South Carolina.

A dedicated teacher and student, Maude updated her education in the care of tuberculosis at the Homer G. Phillips Hospital in St. Louis, Missouri. Never too tired to share her knowledge, she also taught children to read and write. In 1971 she retired from her public health duties and petitioned county officials to start a wellness center for Senior Citizens. The center became a reality in 1980, and Maude worked there, cooking, delivering meals, and picking up seniors who needed transportation. She turned down an invitation from President Reagan to visit the White House, saying, "You can't just call me up and ask me to be somewhere. I've got to do my job."

Maude was the recipient of the following national honors: Outstanding Older South Carolinian Award, 1981; Alexis de Tocqueville Society Award (United Way of America), 1984; Berkeley County Chamber of Commerce's Honorary Citizen's Award; American Institute of Public Service Award, 1984; and an Honorary Doctor of Humanities Degree, Clemsen University, 1983.

Until her death at age ninety-one, she led by example and taught others how community improvement can be accomplished through the efforts of one person.

FOR MAUDE CALLEN: NURSE MIDWIFE, PINEVILLE,
SOUTH CAROLINA, 1951

> I speak of a woman, blue black midwife
> Of April fog, flood, swamp, and July nights
> When Maude Callen's hands layered newsprint
> In circles as a weaver works her loom,
> Slow, to catch blood straw, placenta, save sheets.
> I sing kitchen lamplight, clean cloths, Lysol,
> Cord ties, gloves, gown, and mask; she readies all
> For this crowning, first mother, purple cries.
> I sing of sweat and gush and tear, open thighs
> And triangle moons, ringlets, charcoal hair.
> I sing sixteen-hour days, Maude's tires bare.
> Mud country roads, no man doctor for miles.
> I sing transition, collapse of mountains.
> Crimson alluvium, the son untangled.

HOLDING BACK THE WORLD

for Robert Louis Stauter, M.D.

January in emergency. A girl baby on the gurney.
Terrycloth sleepers, stiff with dried spit-up,
and her mother, a denim globe, pregnant again,
says, *Fever, fever all night long.*

Through our too-big gown, I slide infant fists,
thinking how I love babies, every color like balloons,
they smell of talcum and hope, smile at strangers
wearing white coats and masks. The doctor:

Why the cotton in her ears? The mother, *Roaches.*
My five-year-old got one in her ear so I . . .
Me? A nurse, who pulls the fluff away: cotton, cotton.
He sees puckered canals, angry stuff filling each drum.

Eyes closed, he listens, stethoscope moves shiny as
a quarter on the sidewalk of her small chest.
Deep inside he hears: a wino wheezing on a park bench,
a pot of potato soup bubbling over on the hot plate.

Eyes open. *Sounds like pneumonia, we'll get blood work,*
an x-ray. She'll be admitted. I'll be back.
He's Iowa corn, a silk tie under blue, blue eyes.
This mother never believes men who say they'll return.

It all happened years ago, when I was a young nurse.
And now my grandchildren say I'm mixed up—
no wino ever slept in a baby's chest,
and how could roaches nest in a child's ear?

I was going to say this is a story about
holding back sharp twigs with cotton balls,
how we are happy for what we do not know,
the way you felt before you read this.

$\mathcal{B}$orn in the windy city, Helen Troy remembers moving nearly twenty miles out of
town at age four, where her family lived in a
tent while her father built their new house. "It
was rough on all of us living like that, but life is like
that," Helen recalls. Helen had an appendectomy when
she was ten years old, and she believes this illness, plus the fact that her mother
was a practical nurse, influenced her decision to become a nurse. Immediately
after high school graduation, nineteen-year-old Helen began nurse's training.

She trained and graduated from Mother Cabrini Memorial Hospital in Chicago, Illinois, where there were rules that were strictly enforced. In 1938, "lights
out" was at ten o'clock, but Helen often slipped into the bathroom for late-
night studying. The sisters would knock politely on the bathroom doors and
remind their students it was time for bed. An iron fence surrounded her school
of nursing and, once, Helen got back to the dorm after hours, so her classmates
helped her climb the fence and return to her room before bed check. Since the
school was located in an impoverished area, Helen and her fellow classmates
felt lucky to earn their $4.60 per month; many schools did not pay their stu-
dents. Students worked twelve-hour days, stood when doctors appeared on the
nursing units, and were off duty every other Sunday.

Helen's rich nursing life spans nearly half a century: three years in the U.S.
Army Corps (stateside during World War II due to impaired vision), general

Helen Troy holding Christine, 1959. (Courtesy J. D. Creer, Salem News.*)*

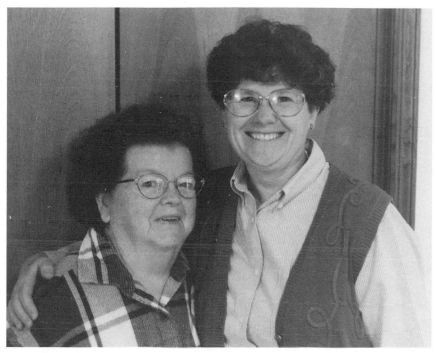

Helen Troy and Jeanne Bryner, 1998. (Courtesy David Bryner.)

duty in Youngstown, Ohio, hospitals, and full-time med-surg staff nurse at Salem Community Hospital for thirty-seven years. Joining the army in 1942, Helen
traveled to Leesville, Louisiana, where she met and married her husband, Tony.
In Louisiana and later at Camp Polk, Texas, she cared for soldiers injured on
maneuvers: "They were getting ready for the real thing, and it was rough."

The mother of three children, Helen continues to be very active in clubs and
volunteer work in her community. She helps with bingo and collects dolls. When
asked if she would again become a nurse, Helen replied, "Not the way things
are today, because you can't give your patients the care they need. There's all the
charting, paperwork, and meetings. Also, I worked hard for my cap, and they
no longer wear them. You can't tell a nurse from a cleaning person nowadays."

LETTER TO CHRISTINE: GIRL BABY FOUND, OHIO
HOSPITAL, 1958

Helen Troy, retired med-surg nurse

Dear Christine: Thanks so much for the wedding picture. You and John
make a handsome pair. I had pearls on my gown also, but it was tea length,

and only my best friend stood up for me. It was war time, the Germans, the Japs. And my mother made our dresses, a cake with banana icing. My Uncle Harold's band played in the basement of St. Sebastian's. Sorry to go on about the old days and the war. It makes everybody sad to look back. There will never be an autumn when I don't think of you. The pink satin dresses on your bridesmaids made me think of your bunting on the cement floor by the boiler room. I swear I can still hear your cry, see your fist waving. Anger is the secret women won't confess later on. It's the broken thing inside us. There's no Peace Corps to fix what's ailing.

People want to help, like me and Flo, two middle-aged nurses headed back to our station after supper. There you were, alone by the elevators in a gray corridor: a new baby in a diaper, your umbilical cord hanging like a ribbon. Of course, we picked you up, carried you like a feather, a shell. The world is filled with crying babies. You know, all those children on the news, Christine, how they look at us, searching, mostly naked? Their arms thin as twigs and stomachs swollen tight as navels hold back a flood of hungers. You know the nuns who come and try to force powdered milk with spoons. We send money, always money. I'm glad you came back, Christine, to look for your roots. Glad you found me and Flo and asked us to tell it all again. We didn't care for that crabby lady from the agency who carried you away one Thursday morning. She had glassy green eyes and a strange smile. And Lord knows what happened to all the flannel gowns and bibs we sewed for you, the bonnets and knit booties the policemen's wives sent. Maybe I told you all the nurses gave up supper breaks to rock you, took turns with your feedings. We even caught Dr. Michaels holding you once. I wanted you to know it all looked different back then, not just the place where they've done away with the stairs and added a whirlpool for rehab. It's all about yielding, Christine, and giving up the question that finally has no right answer. The woman who put you on the floor put you in this world. Try to hold on to that brown-haired boy in the tuxedo and save the ring of flowers in your hair for the days when you fight over the bills, the new sofa, the kids. Step over the fallen leaves, move on, Chris—to your life and the bits of colored paper floating down. Your friend, Helen

Sylvia Engelhardt

$\mathcal{L}$ike many other midcareer nurses, Sylvia Engelhardt works full-time in a busy community hospital while pursuing an advanced degree in allied health. One of the first students to graduate from a two-year associate-degree nursing program, she felt the sting of labels: "I was not a diploma grad." In fact, her first year of college study was not directed toward nursing. She quit after a year, did odd jobs, and couldn't get a sense of direction. "My mother always wanted me to be a nurse; her real vision was for me to be a missionary nurse, but after a year at Bible college, I knew I couldn't do that. I'm a frustrated archeologist, a lover of ancient history who became a nurse."

A longtime member of the Ohio Nurses Association, Sylvia thinks many patients view hospitalization as a pseudo-hotel experience and they become nearly helpless upon admission. "Hand me my tissues; give me my water; I'm hungry, why can't I eat?" She clearly remembers her early days as a nurse when "doctors were Gods and if you wanted to wear a pantsuit, administration inspected you in it beforehand. If you were pregnant, you kept your mouth shut. You wore girdles, jackets, and loose-fitting dresses. We got very creative at hiding our bellies because [if we were known to be pregnant] we were terminated immediately. There was no maternity leave, and seniority was lost. Many nurses had to come back early; they needed the money."

Sylvia remembers that in 1978 the wearing of caps was being challenged;

Sylvia Engelhardt, 1997. (Author's collection.)

though the cap was long a symbol of the nobility of nurses, younger nurses found them nuisances, unclean, and unnecessary. As a personal protest, one of Sylvia's colleagues snipped a piece off her cap daily before she came to work until it was all gone. In the early 1980s most institutions no longer required caps. Still, nurses argued passionately about their disappearance, because the cap was a sort of crown and an integral part of the myth "angels in white." Ask any nurse how she felt the day she was capped and a lump rises in her throat. It worked the same way for other nurses when caps were banished. Sylvia did not feel her nursing skills were tied to wearing a cap.

The mother of two children, Sylvia worked several years on med-surg units and ten years in a chemical dependency unit. At the latter, though patients hid pills and weapons in their underwear and jackets, she was never frightened. When patients cried while Sylvia flushed their pills down the toilet, she reminded them, "You're here to get help." Approximately 25 percent of the patients were put on suicide precautions, and many had to return for a second session of in-house treatment. As a chemical-dependency counselor, she felt her professionalism bloom; she enjoyed one-on-one interaction with patients in recovery from addiction who had suicidal tendencies. "Due to substance abuse, our patients suffered a stunted maturity level. I could talk them down and keep them futuristically focused." Helping her patients work on behavior modification helped her become more centered in her own life. She became a certified chemical dependency nurse; then her hospital was downsized and the unit deemed "unnecessary." Reluctantly, she returned to floor nursing, and, determined to grow professionally, she went back to college. When Sylvia reconnects with former patients who tell her how their lives were changed by the detox program, she feels sad to know such an important community service was eliminated. Given the opportunity, she would not become a nurse again. "We [nurses] are not interchangeable. All nurses should be respected more by the world. Once I get this degree, no one will be able to take it away from me."

HOW I LOST MY JOB AS A STAFF NURSE IN 1969 BECAUSE I WAS PREGNANT

Sylvia Engelhardt, nurse, med-surg unit

> I thought having a baby was the mailman waving
> a letter's good news, the fair's blue ribbon
> for a sweet peach pie. And so, like all women
> I wanted to lean out of my body's white window,

pass ginger cookies to old men and balloons
to toddlers. I forgot to have morning sickness,
to hate my blue jeans and cotton bras for not fastening.
My husband's hands rubbed cocoa butter

across the place my panties covered, a small hotel.
My body had become a bed-and-breakfast for our son.
I found myself smiling over carrots in the grocery,
talking to mothers in the park, walking oddly

and humming over underwear warm from the dryer.
This little story is to say *thank you* to hospital administration
for making me quit in the fifth month,
though we needed my check, we all survived.

AUGUST DELIVERY

What I carried from the Chevy, wet in stiff hospital blankets,
was pink snow in moonlight. There, in my arms, dark hair
soaked in blood smell and placenta was a pilgrim, a tiny dancer,
slant eyes shut tight against this night, this midwife.

Her lips rooted, wanted to suck my full, empty breasts.
Toothless, nameless, folded ears perfect as shells,
a wave had dropped her from a scarlet sea
into the front seat of this world.

Dr. Niemi became a scaffold, eased her skittish mother
to a gurney, while I wrapped feet and fists
delicate as rosettes. I traced her face with the tip
of my finger, she stirred, a pearl, incandescent,

she lay in my cradle until her lungs
brought forth their song,
a small breeze, unafraid.

Part 4

⚜

Heart, do not bruise the breast
That sheltered you so long;
Beat quietly, strange guest.

EDNA ST. VINCENT MILLAY,
"THEME AND VARIATIONS, 2"

Dear Heart: For her science project, my daughter has chosen you. She's asked for my help. Four boxes are on the form. I will need assistance: *some, a little, a lot.* I have a *few* supplies. Her teacher's letter explains the problem need not be large, for example: *think why the family cat claws the sofa.* My daughter is thirteen, the age I was when the Beatles arrived and put girls into screaming fits. The three survivors (George, Paul, Ringo) are making a comeback, though I'm not sure why. Why reinvent the sixties: Kennedy in Jackie's lap, the endless bloody war? My daughter is busy tracing the vena cava; she pauses, *Does it ever stop before we die?* And I'm reaching for answers like a can of pepper on my shelf. I want to tell her about that first dance in the old gymnasium. There was a boy: short, polite, thick glasses. He asked me to slow dance; we moved chest to chest. It made me dizzy, a little short of breath. Something not governed by reason had me, a journey started, and I passed from one place to another. Do you remember, heart, how that sweet boy moved away in July, his father transferred? How you taught me to sacrifice cargo and lighten the ship's load? Heart, please notice how carefully she colors her graph on bypass surgery. *How many attacks can one person have and survive, Mom? I believe it depends on the person and where the damage occurs. Some places in the heart can recover easier, but the heart is never the same. I mean, there's scar tissue forever.* Did you hear that, heart? Look at this science project scattered around the kitchen, books, helpless before the steamy breath of my fried chicken, pages describing your constant bath of warm fluids, the coming in, going out, vessels like ivy vines embracing your pink cottage of four small rooms. You have lived the soft forest, a rose, an apple, radiant in your crimson dress. No prince could reach you, chop you down. Out here, leaves burn. Every day is a torn jacket, worn lapels; wind and sand slap the sclera. We feel the random movement of jaw bones and floor joists. And what have you planned for this child printing her note cards on resuscitation and brain death? Today, I'm wearing my favorite skirt, the one with huge pockets, a wedding band, my navy sweater's on the rocker by the desk, beside my daughter's baby shoes, some paper, this pen. I'm going into the next room to ride the stationary bike, ten minutes or five miles. Be ready, ready for anything; comb your red hair and smile.

Carol L. Johnson

The daughter of a steelworker, Carol L. Johnson has never been afraid of a challenge. Since junior high, she recalls, "I knew that I wanted medicine, I just didn't know which part." Her father always stressed: "You must work hard to get somewhere in life." The first caretaker Carol observed was her grandmother. "My mother was sick; she had some sort of hormonal imbalance, and when she became pregnant at ninety-nine pounds, she'd deliver weighing one hundred and one. We were all premature, and with each pregnancy, the doctors asked my parents, 'If we can only save one of them, who shall it be?' My parents always said, 'Save the baby.'"

A former high school biology and chemistry teacher, Carol walked away from teaching this age group shortly after her students locked her inside a windowless room with no easy way to call for help. Later, she taught pre-nursing students at college who were highly motivated. The first person in her family to obtain a college education, she is passionate about keeping abreast of fast-paced pharmacology changes and high-tech procedures.

Wanting more autonomy in her own career, she invested four years in a master's degree in family primary health care nursing from the University of Pittsburgh to graduate as a nurse practitioner. Slowly, steadily, she has navigated her nursing life's course to become a skilled assistant in the operating room. A cardiothoracic nurse practitioner, Carol harvests the saphenous veins

Carol Johnson, 1998. (Author's collection.)

for open-heart surgeries. "The surgeon told me it would take me two-and-a-half years to feel comfortable taking veins. Then, he asked if I wanted to go to the dog lab or learn on people. I told him I could never hurt an animal."

Realizing the importance of patient education, Carol makes sure pre-operative heart patients understand exactly what will take place in surgery, in recovery, and in cardiac rehab. "I tell them this bone (the sternum) will be cut, leg veins will be taken, and I draw a picture for them. It seems to help. One man did not know his sternum would be cut until I told him. He tore up his consent form and signed out of the hospital against medical advice."

Women face different health challenges. Carol has also worked in women's health and believes sex education should be introduced at younger ages. "Girls are starting their menses at nine or ten now; if we wait until they are twelve or thirteen to educate, it's often too late. They already have a sexually transmitted disease or a baby."

Carol recalls that her worst day of nursing was spent "caring for an ortho-[pedic] patient who was getting ready to go home. She [the patient] threw a fat emboli and died despite ACLS [advanced cardiac life support]. She was in her early forties. I'll never forget it."

Like other nurses, she has formed friendships with some of her patients over the years. One elderly woman (age eighty-two) was very anxious about heart-valve surgery. "She was in good shape otherwise, just a bad valve. We talked and cried together. She decided to put it in the Lord's hands and have the surgery. She did well and lived another seven years."

Carol believes nurses should earn "national certification, the respect of associates and a sense of self-accomplishment and satisfaction." She would definitely become a nurse again, but believes nurses need unions to protect themselves. New nurse practitioners in her facility earn $10,000 to $12,000 more a year than she does. Some of Carol's many honors include membership in the academic honor societies Pi Sigma Pi, Tri Beta, Delta Epsilon Sigma, and Sigma Theta Tau, and she is listed in *Who's Who in American Nursing*.

ON MY GLOVES BLOOD DRIES IN A PATTERN LIKE FADED
ROSES IN WALLPAPER

Carol Johnson, cardiothoracic nurse practitioner

A man's draped body hovers, a green airplane
Above the floor, his chest pried open, an old
Pantry door. I harvest saphenous veins,

My knife splits legs, mid-thigh to ankle, in cold
Rooms where many hearts are afraid for one.
I snip the soft red, lift quivering pink casing.
Wipe with red dishrags, nurses' work never done.
A catheter inside the vein, fluids racing
Through. The surgeon passes a length of black string.
This much, he says. Carefully, I cut the fresh
Wafer the body has given up. Bring
My half-moon needle down and up through flesh.
A secret embroidery, I have learned to close,
To comfort the leg oozing, mourning its loss.

AT DUSK, TWO WOMEN TRACE A HEART'S RIVER

My friend Leona follows me into the medicine room.
Her story opens like a meadow's bosom aching with thorns.
In the time it takes this nurse to mix a pain shot,
Leona explains her mother's old heart:

The doctor says it's like a cabin, too many winters,
all rooms flooding, timbers soft as melon.
She knows the black lightning will strike again and again
until raven wings replace the sky.

Leona says her West Virginia mother fainted Sunday
in K-Mart, the row between baby clothes and shovels,
her brown tweed skirt gathered like roots
around gnarled knees and her skin nestled dew

Beside us, a cupboard door slams,
but instead of warm bread, we smell
the hospital's belly, instead of porch shade,
fevered metal lights. At dusk, two women trace

a heart's river down eighty blue-ribbon summers.
For a few minutes, chores wait, we stand
in the doorway's rain, speak of sorrow
and blackberries, wipe stained hands

on gingham aprons
push stray hairs from our eyes
breathe the night air,
knowing we are halfway home.

Jeanette Price

A tiny woman who stood five-foot two and weighed just one hundred pounds, Jeanette Price was born to a harpist and a homemaker in 1883 in Aberdaire, Wales. Her family moved to the coal-mining community of Scranton, Pennsylvania, when she was a toddler. By the time Jeanette was six years old, both of her parents were dead. Her mother died giving birth to her fifth sister, and different Welsh families in Scranton adopted Jeanette and each of her sisters. Raised separately, the sisters continued to speak the language of their birthplace while learning English. Even though they lived with different families, they came together as siblings occasionally, and one formal photograph even documents the faces of these six teenage sisters in their Sunday dresses.

Near the end of her high school years, Jeanette's adopted father died, and shortly after, her adopted mother started drinking heavily. When her adoptive-family brothers and sisters visited, they realized Jeanette deserved better surroundings. Financially able to provide her with a fine opportunity, they sent her to Ann Arbor, Michigan, for nursing school. She was the only girl in her birth family to obtain a professional education. After graduating in 1908 she remained at the Michigan hospital where she'd trained; when World War I started, she enlisted immediately as an army nurse. In October 1918 she sailed for France and Base Hospital 114 at Beauderet, six miles from Bordeaux.

Jeanette Price, 1915. (Courtesy Esther Gundry.)

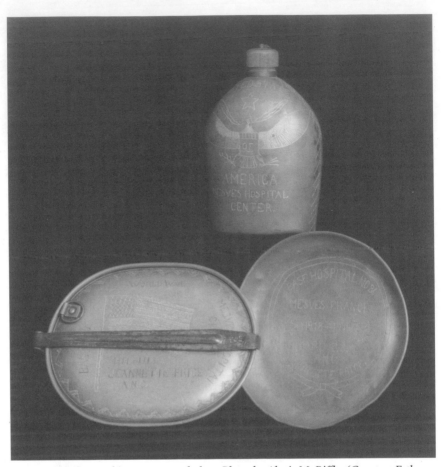

Jeanette Price's mess kit, canteen, and plate. Photo by Alexis M. Riffle. (Courtesy Esther Gundry.)

Here she and her colleagues worked eighteen-hour shifts caring for the wounded, fevered, and dying soldiers transported from surrounding battle-fields. In Bordeaux, juxtaposed against the horrors of war, she saw wonderful monuments and castle ruins surrounded by moats. After draining shifts in the fracture ward, she took walks and observed women washing their clothes in the river. No doubt the small French villages dotted with wooden carts traveling narrow streets were romantic. She corresponded with former patients who were transferred to Walter Reed Hospital and noted their deaths in her photograph album. She fell ill with the flu and was hospitalized in France, and although she survived, her heart sustained damage and her stamina never returned.

Discharged from the Army in 1920 Jeanette continued hospital nursing in Mineoloa, New York; Huntington, West Virginia; and Dayton, Ohio; where bed-side nurses were in demand. Her small home in Glenburn, Pennsylvania, reflected her love for decorating with linens and curtains she had sewn. The leatherbound photo album she left behind is very telling about her life in France and the men who were her "charges." She comments on the soldiers as "plucky, brilliant, and those who made the supreme sacrifice." Several of the photos are rows of quiet white crosses.

In September 1929, at age forty-six, despite her weakened condition, she marched with other veteran nurses in a large American Legion parade in Pennsylvania and died the next day. At her funeral taps were played, and a one-armed World War I veteran took charge of the firing squad.

LETTER TO WORLD WAR I SURGEON DR. HENRY RUSSELL, FROM NURSE JEANETTE PRICE, SEPTEMBER 1929

My dearest Henry,

You were the pluckiest surgeon and able to talk me through those convulsing scarlet boys screaming before and after the ether. Those men shot in the belly, who'd die in four days anyway, smelling putrid as rotting fish, begging to be done with it, vomiting black into our white enamel pans. Men who'd kiss their widows' photo and curse the general's clean hands pinning medals to their sheets. We all knew only the dying receive the cross.

Many seasons of grapes and wheat and hay have passed, and I have kept our story inside me like a prisoner. As we are now between worlds and oceans, you must think me daft to write this letter. Oh Henry, France was beautiful and ugly in war. We were so young, and it is easy to be caught on hope's barbed wire. I know you didn't want to leave. That awful cough. That flu. I suppose God was angry too.

Remember the village by the river and your barber's fine, tall son? How Pascal dressed the boy in knickers those last years, hoping to save him from the front? He left for the trenches. Five months in a field hospital. The Red Cross wrote to Pascal: *no arms, no legs, no eyes.* Pascal sent hundreds of francs to buy the wooden arms and legs his boy would need. He is home now; a black scarf covers his raw sockets and the fat, flat nose a surgeon built him sits above his two new lips. Most of his teeth are gone. He can eat. He is able to say over and over, "Kill me Papa, please kill me."

Forgive me for not standing at your rainy grave; the flu pressed me to my sheets. I am very tired today and dreamed your voice last night. The valves in my heart are damaged, and that is the reason I cannot sweep and dust in the same day. Though the nursing director wrote many times on my behalf, I was never able to visit Wales.

Today, we march in a parade for veterans. Sarah, who worked all those months with me in the fracture ward, will not be there, nor James nor Thomas, our orderlies. Do you remember them, Henry? Tromping thick mud in, their stretchers dripping blood? Are they with you, Henry? And where is that? I have settled in a small Pennsylvania town near my sister and her children. It's not the Paris life we both wanted then, when there was no end to the barking guns and no moment to sit on the lilac porch of love's house. I shall wear your ring forever. Jenny

Part 5

These scars, I tell myself, are learned.

EAVAN BOLAND, "BRIGHT-CUT IRISH SILVER"

Nora Mary Carmody McNicholas

$\mathcal{B}$orn March 29, 1909, in Liscarrol, County Cork, Ireland, Nora Mary Carmody McNicholas vividly recalls how at fourteen she rode the Cedric through December's fierce weather on her voyage to America. Bound for a new country and a new life, she was constantly seasick and lost twenty pounds during the crossing. Nora admits, "I prayed for the ship to sink; I was so sick; I vomited and vomited; it was cold and I was frightened by the high waves." One of the youngest passengers on the ship, she remembers how very disconnected she felt from home and at the same time, how lucky that she, at least, understood the English language.

Once on Ellis Island, she was afraid to go to sleep with a person on the bunk above her because she had never seen a legless bed or slept in one. Her older sister had traveled to America two years ahead of her, and Nora went to live with her in a small apartment in Brooklyn. Like many other Irish immigrants, Nora was reluctant to answer questions in school because of her brogue. Her first job was as a file clerk for Brooks Brothers at 44th and Madison in downtown New York.

Nora met her husband, James, at an Irish dance; they were married fifty-six years and had three children. When her youngest son was twelve years old, Nora decided she should not sit idly at home. At fifty, she returned to school to study nursing. Her husband totally supported this decision, but her in-laws thought she wasn't intelligent enough to pass her coursework. Nora graduated in one year from the YWCA School for Practical Nurses in Brooklyn and spent six years working a med-surg unit at King's Park Hospital, a privately owned hospital in

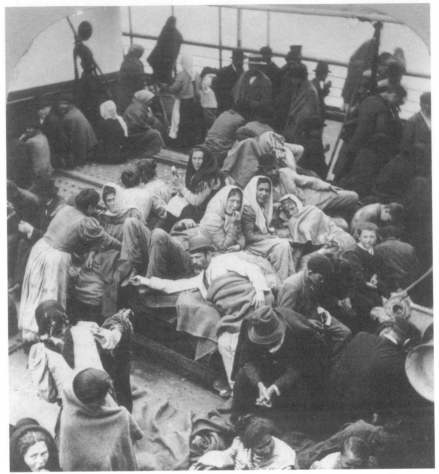

Emigrants coming to the "land of promise," 1920. (Courtesy Library of Congress.)

Brooklyn. She ended her nursing career with eight years of private duty nursing. This gentle Irish woman, who embraced living and learning, died July 4, 2001.

WHAT IT COST TO CROSS THE ATLANTIC

Nora Carmody McNicholas, retired private duty nurse

Born Celtic and poor, small girls learned to knit
In school; Miss Scriven taught the price of loved land.
Fathers plowed space, dug coal, or broke bricks.
Christmas treats were crackers tied to tree branches.
Some war blew out our castle's brave heart,

Stone steps, so steep, led nowhere but the sky.
We played there, counting thatched roofs until dark,
Didn't know mother's bloody cough meant she'd die.
Kathleen Culhane was my best friend's name.
I'd write her later about my hard trip,
Landing at Ellis Island, papers lost, shame.
An angry man walked me back to my ship.
Fourteen, alone, ten days of winter's waves
So sick, nothing stayed inside but Ireland.

Jeanne Bryner

$\mathscr{T}$he middle child in a family of six, I am
the first person in my family to obtain a professional education. A graduate of Trumbull
Memorial Hospital School of Nursing in Ohio
and Kent State University's Honors College, I have
worked as a waitress, babysitter, motel maid, and fac-
tory worker prior to becoming a nurse. All of these jobs have helped prepare
me for the challenge of emergency-room nursing. I believe family illness
definitely influenced my career selection: My mother had manic-depressive illness; my father was an alcoholic; and my youngest brother has cerebral palsy. I
grew up with brothers and sisters; somebody always needed a hug or a bath, a
blanket or a band-aid. Those people were not always children.

Having the opportunity for a college education, I witnessed women who
had achieved self-actualization, and I hungered for it. Until I became a nursing
student at age twenty-five, I had never volunteered or worked inside a hospital.
I found bedside care was as familiar as breathing. It was dying I had never seen,
and the different faces of pain, the unpredictable ways our lives become tangled
during illness. Ignorance about the difficulty of chemistry and science allowed
me to plunge head first into a world of giving and receiving messages and medicines for curing all manner of ailments.

I have worked med-surg units, pediatrics, IV team, intensive care, emergency, and urgent care, this last for three years. Many of my experiences dealing

Author, 2003. (Courtesy Gary Harwood.)

with patient care moved my heart's pen to poetry. It was the encouragement of my husband and college professors that sent me back to college for a degree in English. Ten years later, I graduated. I had no idea a person getting an English degree would need four semesters of Spanish. Several fine women served as my mentors: Betsy Hoobler, Gloria Young, Vivian Pemberton, and Maggie Anderson. My writing life, my sense of fulfillment for what that life provides, would certainly have turned out differently had they not offered me guidance and friendship.

My fondest memory in nurse's training was graduation because my entire family was present; even though my mom was dead, she had the best seat in the house. Though I realize there are many problems in the field of nursing, I have never dreaded going to work and would become a nurse again. Nurses do not earn salaries commensurate with their responsibilities and educational requirements, and this issue is as old as the profession.

A strong believer in the healing power of language, I teach community writing workshops in schools, universities, senior citizen facilities, and cancer support groups.

BECOMING A NURSE

My arms lift up as this drunk man stumbles
toward me. He claims to be an FBI informant,
demands two x-rays and the truth
about Kennedy's assassination.

I can barely keep my balance in this dance.
He circles our emergency room, a broken boat
cursing the moon. This far inland
we cannot hear the gull's cry or feel the wave's fist,

but I can see his family: four sleepy toddlers
clinging to a hollow woman harnessed to him
in her wrong-buttoned dress. We are all in motion,
and the bow aches under our weight.

It exhumes my smashed tea set, mama's bloodied lip,
little girls learning that women must clean up
earth's magma, the kinetics of sweeping linoleum
after the bomb, the pressure of hunger and combat.

This is the way the heart pulls forward
to our life's work. We embrace something endless,
like sand. We wash and floss the wrecked ship's hull
and its seedy sailors who are always arriving on our island.

BREATHLESS

Dear Trent, today I was remembering the clay faces of parents pulling red
wagons in Akron's pediatric hospital and a three-year-old girl named Ashley
with a brain tumor the size of a melon, that pale train of four-year-old boys
pushing their IV poles like Sisyphus with his rock day after day. Maybe you
can't recall me, the fumbling nursing student with hazel eyes, gripping her
pink spiral notebook, who mixed enzymes in your applesauce. You drew
me a picture that July 1978. And it was splendid too: your mommy in her
jeans and gingham blouse, her boyfriend, Luke, on his Harley, the one
Mommy rode on weekends when she missed visiting, and your beagle, Sam,
wagging his tail by a single blue flower. You handed it to me, pointing wildly
with your clubbed nails: *That's my dog, Sam. And that's my house. That's
where I live. Here, keep it.* It was awfully cold that summer, and you didn't
tell me what to do with this painting you left behind. Please listen. The oaks
in my neighbor's pasture are awash today with autumn's blush, and on some
island, sandaled monks are praying for war orphans, and me, I cradle almost everything: my daughter's baby tooth, the smell of apple fritters in my
granny's kitchen, this faded manila paper filled with crayola marks. In the
next room, Kenny G is playing "Breathless" on his sax. Wherever you are,
Trent, come sit with me in his horn's amazing shade. I know now it's wrong
to want more than this scrap of paper, sinful to rescue angels.

BODY OF KNOWLEDGE: REMEMBERING DIPLOMA
SCHOOLS, 1976

Where have I put the silver bandage scissors
they told me never to lose, my student name tag,
the snowy candle I carried for the capping ceremony?

Where are the showers' lathered girls, naked, laughing?
What's become of our housemother bent over
crossword puzzles night after night?

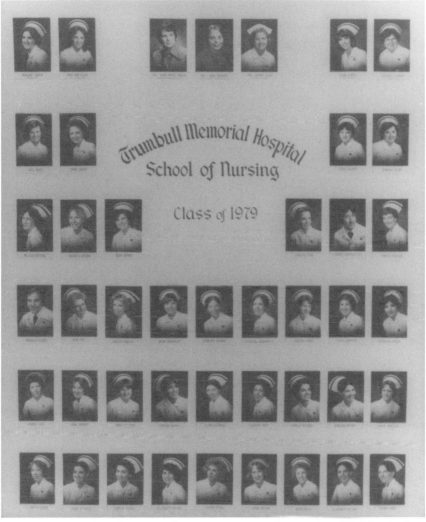

Trumbull Memorial Hospital School of Nursing, 1979 graduates. Photo by Abbey Studio.
(Author's collection.)

Where is Louise Frye, who ran out one autumn day screaming:
I can't be a nurse. Where is her father's Texaco shirt
and their sorry station wagon?

What were their names? Those two girls who got ulcers
their junior year, and the one with glasses who died
from *leukemia*—that beautiful, beautiful word.

Gone are the thousand days our professors stood
patient, in ochre suits and wrote like cave painters,
something about pathways from the brain to the heart,
wanted us to remember.

LETTER FROM WARD THREE

I.

I am busy today watching my ceiling crack grow
green plaster. My hands fold over the collapsed
melon of my womb; this is where my five babies
floated like pink letters in a mailbox. I remember
doctors in the delivery rooms, postured shells
in olive gowns, slapping the child until he found
his voice like a fingernail against the blackboard.
They are all that became of me, ribbons and shoelaces
that bind me to corners of the rooms where it rains
yellow trees and paper cranes beat their wings,
forgetting where it is they wanted to fly.

II.

I had some nice things once: a wedding band,
lavender stationery, a black lace slip. I could put
clothespins in my mouth, taste the clean wood,
and hang diapers in neat rows.
My fingers sifted darkness like sand on the beach.
Maybe you think I will die,
I am weightless as an old movie on the screen. I urge
myself back over and over through steel wires like miners
feeling their way through tunneled cave-ins.
I am harmless as the back door of a valley,
quiet as a gray plowhorse pacing these unclean tiles.

III.

There's a tide storm rising in the gulf. Thinking back,
I forget the man's face buried among the babies,
the owner of giant fists, the climbing on and off,
the milkman's sandy smile, my broken picture of Jesus.
Blood on both sides of my table, winter, a piano with no song.
Naturally, I believe the boats will come for me,

or I would never invent footsteps falling close in the night.
Once, I was young, a woman with enormous eyes,
the thing about living is hesitation, the snowflakes saying your name,
the leaves gossiping, and the sun telling you
it is easy—that bread is better than hay,
that everything that needs you is real.

Avanell Arlene Sutherland

$\mathscr{A}$ farm girl from Coalburg, Ohio, Avanell Arlene Sutherland seemed to have a natural gift for helping and healing, so her family was never surprised she chose nursing for her life's work. Her parents' third child, born in August 1927, she was a participant in the cycles of planting and harvesting, living and dying. While yet a youngster, she performed her first surgical procedure when the family cat's leg collided with a mowing machine and was nearly amputated. Knowing the cat's limb was beyond saving, Arlene completed the amputation, bandaged the wound tightly and faithfully cared for the cat, who healed well and lived several years, running around the farm on three legs.

When she was in high school, she traveled by train with other family members to a New York hospital where her brother was a patient after being wounded in Iwo Jima. Without a doubt, seeing her brother being well cared for by nurses and physicians helped steer her career choice. After high school, she immediately went to train at Ohio's Youngstown Hospital Association of Nursing, where she was affectionately known to her classmates as "Johnnie." Training was a world filled with early rising and long hours of studying, textbooks and lectures, new friends and new challenges. Her farm background had prepared Arlene well for the arena of scholarship.

She served early nursing assignments in emergency rooms in Ohio, New Jersey, Virginia, and Florida. Her family remembers one nurse story she told

Arlene "Johnnie" Johnson, nursing graduation, 1948. (Courtesy Joann Johnson.)

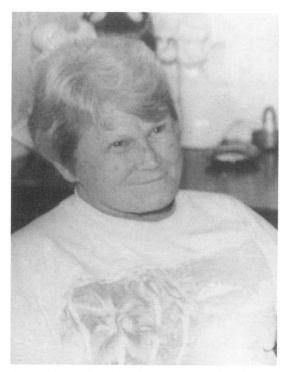

Arlene Johnson Sutherland, retired, 1986. Photo by
Phyllis Fischer. (Courtesy Joann Johnson.)

several times over the years about an assault incident: a man was stabbed in his
head with a huge field knife. When Arlene was taken to see him, the patient was
still awake and talking! The knife had miraculously missed all vital vessels; it
was a rare injury to behold, even for a farm girl.

While working in the southern region of the United States, Arlene witnessed
segregated healthcare delivery. In some communities, white patients and black
patients were admitted to separate hospitals. Arlene became a skilled surgical
nurse, and—when she returned to Ohio and found no openings for emergency-
room nurses—a firm surgical instructor.

She saved at least three of her own family members through her nursing
care: her husband, after a severe electrical shock; a nephew, after a near drowning; and at a family gathering, a child who was choking on candy was spared
due to her quick intervention.

An avid gardener and cook, she had a cabin in the Pennsylvania mountains
where she could enjoy another favorite pastime: reading. She was fond of auc-
tions and garage sales, traveled to Alaska and the New England states, and nearly
moved to Maine so she could be closer to lighthouses. Retired less than ten
years, she was diagnosed with lung cancer in December 1992, and eight weeks

later she died in her home surrounded by family. Arlene's lifelong motto was, "Always do what will hurt the least amount of people."

LOVING WOMEN

for Arlene Sutherland, surgical nursing instructor

Dear Arlene: So much time has passed since you explained how germs move about the OR, not with wings like butterflies, but on dust particles and a sneeze. I think of November's early Sunday morning, how we unfolded green sterile drapes, wrong, in triangles, like bandannas for an outlaw's face, how we all laughed, nervous students in scrubs. I didn't know then science was so hard, everything bound to scalpels. You were right about the surgeons: they never thought anything was funny. It was amazing to learn nurses could pass silence like instruments with their eyes, a curved needle looked exactly like the moon's spine, and the red vault of the body was so much like an apple, growing soft at its heart. I wish now I'd been a better talker. When I see purple, I always feel sad, like this berry stain on my daughter's blouse. Sometimes I want to cry over the plums stacked in the market. They look so much like my mother's eyes. Lines of purple were painted on your forehead the last time I saw you, sleepy against white sheets in bed. Do you see what I mean? I was thirty-eight and wanted to say thank you for helping me with part of my life. But your sisters were there by the flowers, the daffodil's slow jazz horn, the blue sea in your eyes. It came out all wrong, like a three-year-old reading a dictionary. I know purple is not the color of love; it's all anger and pain, a chalice without wine, a woman with her tongue cut out.

THIS RED OOZING

I'm a nurse in emergency.
You're a hostess at Benny's Lounge,
thirty-five, divorced. After three beers,
you can never let the friend of a friend
drop you off at your apartment,
then ask him in for coffee.

Never pee with an accountant in the house,
especially one dragging his briefcase.
See, how the balding sheriff shakes
his *I-told-you-so eyes*

while you tell how the man shoved
your bathroom door open,
pulled out his revolver, grinned.

We know what he said next, we hear it
nearly every week: *I'm gonna fuck you;*
you scream, I'll kill you.
We believe you cried, begged on knees,
told him your kids might be home soon.
You kneeling on the fuzzy pink rug—
he likes that—you genuflecting.

The safety clicks on his forty-five.
You know guns; your father hunted—
black roundness against your right temple,
your hoop earrings clang, train whistles
in your ears and his words squeeze:
suck hard, bitch.

We're sorry, but now the doctor
makes you say all of it again,
how a single lamp burns on the nightstand
and your kids smile in their school pictures.
How tightly he holds the cold muzzle to your neck,
jerks your dark hair like a mane and rips
you until you bleed, your breath becomes
grunts, your face in a pillow.

Doctors in the ER speak like priests,
and they try to explain it, clean it up
when they swab, hunting for sperm, trying
to mount rage on slides—dead or alive.

This red oozing,
this trail from your buttocks to your thighs
will not fill him, and it doesn't matter
how many times you throw up green
or call on God or bruises rise
like small irises on your cheekbones,
the razor moves on.

The friend of your friend
with the pinstriped suit will probably walk.
I think you know that.
What you don't know is how he rapes you
endlessly: how he crawls out of your lipstick
tube in the morning, slithers out of the soapy
washcloth in the shower, snickers every Friday
when you dust those photos on your stand.
How his boots climb the back stairs
of your mind year after year
as he comes and comes and comes.

THE LABOR OF TENDERNESS

Dear Mom: Yesterday I took my daughter, your granddaughter, to work. I'm a registered nurse now, twenty-one years. With my own money I bought her a shirt, an olive vest with covered buttons, and wheat-colored trousers with French seams. Her shoes cost $20.00 (on sale). And yes, you're probably right about me spoiling her, but she's my daughter. She shouldn't traipse around the emergency room in faded jeans and dirty sneakers. Her hair is the same color as yours: it is the color of honey. She was able to take temperatures with a computerized thermometer. Yeah, Mom, the numbers click so fast it makes the patient dizzy to watch, then there's a beep like a bird singing somewhere. She was beside me for twelve hours, the entire day. It wasn't exactly like summer days in the small yard with you—handing clothespins, hoping the wind would pick up and the rain would hold off until the last load. But I tried to lead her easy. She was close and warm and eager to please. Something like those first few times you lifted me to hang diapers and dad's red hankies. When the first man came with a swollen ankle, I helped her make an ice bag. We have plastic bags covered with white cloth, Mom. And crushed ice falls neatly from a silver machine. It wasn't like Sunday morning and me emptying stale bread from a sack, me climbing the gray chair to fetch fresh ice for your black eyes. It wasn't like digging through the junk drawer for a gum band to tie the sack off like an umbilical cord. No, it was neat and clean, and there were four white ties to secure it. She watched me order x-rays when I suspected a fractured navicular. Mom, I even know how to spell *navicular*. And it's OK to order x-rays. I do that. Before any doctor looks at the patient, I make a decision. Alone. And my daughter was with me. She palpated pulses on either side of a wrist. In the afternoon, I showed her how to set the wheelchair's brakes, how to steer a person without hurting them, how to avoid sharp turns and go slow. Mom, a lady came in vomiting, and she gave her a basin. She said, *Ma'am here's a chair, please have a seat.* She was gentle as a stewardess. It was nothing like a week of five kids having the flu in one bedroom. The vomit glistened and was a similar green, but it was so civilized and orderly; and nobody was weeping over the mess. Mom, she saw a man with his finger nearly cut off from a factory accident. And her voice was clear and soft when she told him: *My Dad has one cut off too.* Yes, some things here are the same: the children in our valley are still learning their fathers' body must be given up. But, Mom, she believes in her father, believes he's a mountain, wants to go to work with him next year. She has blue eyes, Mom, not anything like your brown. And remember how story problems gave me hives? She does algebra with a pen. Mom, we wish you were here; we're having a great time. We're doing all right. Your girls are fine. We're just so damn fine.

AFTER THE BATTLE: IN A ROOM WHERE WE HAVE TRIED TO SAVE A LIFE

The curtain is pulled and it is time to lift the oxygen
from the nose; be careful of the hair's cilia.
I hurry to turn off hissing of hoses and machines.
I have been here before,

wetting a white cloth for the face, sliding down
the jaw's crease and landing in a neck filling
slowly with lavender. I am lost in a glacier
of glistening spittle and the mouth

surprised in an "O." I am afraid of the undressing,
how the arms straighten for a gown of blue flowers.
I have been here before,
washing the hands of a man and thinking of my children

on busy August days. Falling, falling. There is not time
to clean out all the palms hold. The black wheels turn
as I wipe gel from the rib cage and trace a burn mark
on the chest. I want to kiss it. I want to kiss it.

Once, long ago, I would know where to gather roots
for a poultice, how to kneel and be forgiven.
Another face enters the room, a woman.
Together we roll this trunk, these four limbs.

I have been here before.
Sour breath of warm stool mushrooms inside the buttocks.
I hear the sound of running water and throw
the body's mud away.

A final sigh or moan comes after this.
It is the wind and not a complaint. There is a strange land
ahead. Here, take this pillow for its dreams.
I am afraid, so I talk about rain and a trip

we may take to Scotland—how the grass is tall there
and the music pure. The man's journey has started,
and I'm looking to see if I can tell anything about the road.
I have lost something

in the business of heart scribbles and paper strips
curled upon this floor. I toss them like confetti.
Once, long ago, the needles were swords
and the man was a knight, maybe a king.

His blood meant battles for a god, for honor, a country.
His spirit is a hawk circling. I have been here before
crying, picking up heads on the moor
knowing it is done.

Part 6

Who are those who suffer?
I do not know, but they call to me.

PABLO NERUDA, "THE MOUNTAIN AND THE RIVER"

BUTTERFLY

The thing I keep thinking is these young men
are much too weak to make love. These boys
with yellow hair and blue tattoos and bristly
mustaches who are married and dying with AIDS

cannot enter each other in the old way—bony hips hang,
unbeautiful, too tired to pump. Like soft cow bells
their hoop earrings tinkle in ER, room thirteen,
as they press cool cloths to foreheads, pass tissues

for sticky green phlegm. They wait for the doctor
and lab techs and nurses who mark their plastic name bands
with a *B*. *B* for *blood hazard*. *B* for *boys*. *B* for *bad*.
Orange-ball stickers tag their charts, flags go up that say danger.

I am their nurse, and when they ask for blankets,
they cover each other the way I spread quilts
on my daughter in her crib. They are half a butterfly
on gray cement, their skin shrinks and tarnishes,

bodies cave in, revival tents collapsing the final week
of summer. They cough as I enter their room,
and something in me stiffens. Even this far away
in my mask and gown and gloves trying hard to say—*I care*

that you suffer, that your cottage burns—its flames
reach inside my tent. Whatever chokes in this fire is large
and soundless and pale. I keep thinking as these men lift
each others' heads from the pillow, gently tilt straws

close to dusky lips, hold hands as needles dig for veins
and pull and straighten hospital sheets hour after wounded hour—
they are migrating back to the cocoon, the place
where brown masks protect the unbeautiful.

Genevieve Schmitt

*W*orld War II veteran nurse First Lieutenant Genevieve Schmitt recalls, "I had no inclination to become a nurse. I wanted to be a teacher, but my best friend chose nursing." Pursuing an education meant leaving her family and hometown, so why not stay close to a friend? A 1929 graduate of St. John's Hospital School of Nursing in Cleveland, Ohio, she spent most of her nursing life in public health positions, first in Ohio, later in Michigan: "I was responsible for eight districts in Cleveland; I had my own secretary. I liked working for cities because you get a good pension, honey." Later, she received a scholarship and another degree from Case Western Reserve. "There are letters I can write behind my name, and I think it means I'm a certified public health nurse. You know, I just can't remember everything."

Having been stationed near Worcestershire, England, during the war, she vividly recalls England's bombed-out appearance, "like someone had taken a huge wrecking ball to the buildings." At age thirty-six, she was older than most of the nurses in her unit, and they frequently looked to her for comfort. To the young nurses, England was a country of dampness, quaint pubs, latrines, and cold-water bathing. "I spent two years and four months overseas. I saw Piccadilly Circus and 10 Downing Street. I visited Scotland and saw Carnegie's home. For ten dollars, I bought a bicycle and tried to learn how to ride it; I had long legs and I thought they'd do for brakes. I got rid of it [the bicycle] after a week."

Genevieve Quinn Schmitt, age 92, 1997. (Author's collection.)

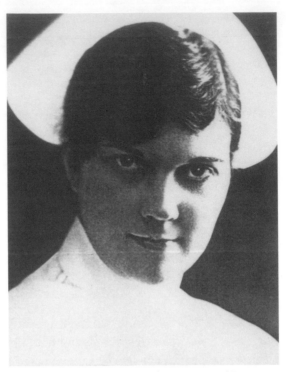

Genevieve Quinn, nursing graduation, 1929. (Courtesy Sisters of Charity of St. Augustine, Richland, Ohio.)

Remembering her traumatized soldiers, Genevieve says, "In your own life, you choose what you want to do. In the army, you do what they say." Several Italian soldiers were among her patients, and one of them filigreed her metal drinking cup. "I thought to never lose it [the cup], but then, I never imagined I'd live to be ninety-two. Things get lost over the years." She reports, "All our doctors were the very best; one of them, a Jewish doctor, created an ear. I mean, a person looks funny with only one ear, so it made the wounded man look better, more normal."

Genevieve's commanding officers chose a space for the nurses and soldiers to socialize and rest when off duty. The "Fallen Arches" tent became a place of solace and some fun where the nurses and doctors would put on skits and have a beer. When asked what makes a good nurse, she said, "I'm from the old school; nurses should be kind and listen. They need to pretend the patient is related to them: their sister or mother." The proud recipient of the Military Order of the Purple Heart, Genevieve slowly smokes her cigarette and says, "Did you know I'm going blind? I used to drive a Monte Carlo. I loved that car. Oh yes, I'd become a nurse again."

MENTALLY TRAUMATIZED UNIT, NURSING ASSIGNMENT, ENGLAND 1942

Genevieve Schmitt, retired first lieutenant, U.S. Army

The road back is a barn filled with glazed men
Night bombs, pieces fly off under heavy fire.
They went screaming beneath their beds, pale hens
Hiding from a fox, caught on crimson wire.
What is war but a spear of wood driven
Into a wall for men to be nailed to it?
Village dawns of raped women given
As field rations, grandmothers shot and split.
What did I know then of street gallows?
Bullets gouging another man's soft thickness?
A young nurse brings her smile to swallow
Like a pill, as if blown minds are the sickness.
Two years, I walked among these ruins, stunned
And saw where the cleaver's plunge left no stain.

Phyllis Fischer

A carpenter's daughter and Ohio native, Phyllis Fischer faced career choices when the selection was limited for women. Realizing how much her parents wanted her to have a professional education was only one side of future's graph. Accepted professional paths for women included becoming a teacher, librarian, secretary, clerk, or nurse. A shy person, she believes, "If someone told me when I was in school that I should become a teacher, I would have fainted on the spot." Though her mother insisted she take speech, every debate made her break out in a cold sweat. At the end of high school, "being a librarian seemed dull, though now, I do not think so." A graduate of City Hospital in Cleveland, Ohio, and a BSN (bachelor of science, nursing) graduate of Western Reserve University in 1950, she was in the first class to follow the nurse Cadet Corps.

Rich memories of her fine grade school teachers and their lessons have stayed with her these many years. "I learned more in grade school than anywhere else. My teachers were friendly and dedicated. During the war, we had air raid drills, and Miss Anderson wheeled the piano in while another teacher led us singing *The Beer Barrel Polka*. Also, we gathered around the radio to hear the King of England abdicate his throne." As children, Phyllis and her brother often had bronchitis. "Mother rubbed stuff on my chest, and we had to drink onion soup."

Phyllis remembers there were twenty-one students in her nursing class and

Phyllis Fischer, 1998. (Author's collection.)

ex-army nurses served as instructors. "They were very organized and demanded excellence in learning procedures. I was very impressed with them." She recalls the high ceilings, high windows, metal bed, and dresser of her dorm room, which "looked just like a detention home from the movies." There were cockroaches everywhere—large ones. Knowing a nurse's duty meant long hours and little rest, her director advised them, "Don't push yourself until you drop. When you are the only nurse responsible for all these patients, you must take care of yourself. If you care for them until you drop, they will have no one." Phyllis never forgot this valuable message.

Phyllis served as a staff nurse, head nurse, and supervisor before spending twenty-four years in nursing education. Every new class of nursing students had its own personality and sense of community. "It was an accident that I became a teacher, but I loved the students and learned from them constantly," she says.

She is very thankful for her medical knowledge because it has helped her select care for herself and family members. She readily explains, "I liked helping people; it helped in my personal growth." However, in her opinion, the exhausting duties of nursing have not changed much in the last fifty years, and this troubles her greatly. "Airplane pilots and truck drivers cannot legally work beyond certain hours because sleep deprivation impairs judgment; yet hospitals require long hours, mandatory overtime, and working an evening shift followed by days. Hospitals hire a part-time nurse without benefits and require him or her to frequently work the fifth day [forty hours]. Nurses are taught and prepared to do many more things than the hospital allows them to do because the hospital does not provide sufficient staff, and the patient is short changed." Phyllis hopes nurses' unions will help "rectify these conditions, including identifying the amount of staff necessary to care for a specific number of patients with a certain acuity." Busy with photography, tole painting, embroidery, and yard work, Phyllis enjoys every minute of retirement.

TO MY TOWN CAME A SNOW STORM, NURSE'S DIARY, CITY HOSPITAL OF CLEVELAND, OHIO, NOVEMBER 24, 1950

Phyllis Fischer, retired nursing instructor

Out of nowhere, our city was buried in tons of snow.
On 6 West, only Alma and I (an aide, a nurse)
Make it in. Thirty-two patients on our floor.
The dietitian brings food in huge pots,
Big spoons to ladle eggs and oats in bowls.

Call lights twinkling like Christmas-tree bulbs.
If we weren't so busy, I'd tell you more.
Morning talk's a wagon carrying basins, soap,
Towels to each bed. Our hands are the patron saints
Of forward motion. Here, read the newspaper:

A woman expecting her fourth baby was pulled by sled
to E. 152nd St. A police ambulance took her to Glenville.
Isolated persons are to display signals in the snow: an "I"
means medical aide; an "F" means fire or food.
Fifty-four boy scouts had to be rescued by tanks & trucks
& an airplane on skis in the dusk and night.
140 stranded workmen at Jones & Laughlin Steel are being
fed by Red Cross Workers. At St. Luke's the lights were out
from 9:45 A.M. until 7:00 P.M. A thirty-ton Sherman tank
clanked through the Memorial Shoreway to help 50 motorists.
A bakery truck stalled in a drift, set up shop, and sold out
in minutes. Four men have died today shoveling snow.
The mayor asks milk purchases be restricted to babies,
children, and the sick. Streetcars are motionless. One C.E.I.
worker walked 7 hours from E. 28th to Public Square to work.
Olivia DeHaviland tours U.S. and Canada in "Romeo & Juliet."
Governor Frank J. Lausche declares a state of emergency.
Thirty taxis from the Yellow Cab Co. marooned about the city.
Police captains issue warning to looters, "Shoot to Kill."
While there is an ample supply of coal, delivery is impossible.

Alma passes fresh water, takes temps. Me? I take pulses.
Think one patient at a time: Is the wound red? Draining?
Give pain shots, change bloody dressings and top sheets.
Joined together, two women become the horse
Answering bells, lifting, turning pale faces inside sick gowns
While firemen prop the Electric Sweeper Service Co. roof

Sagging under the snow's weight. We drag sweaty linen
Bags to metal chutes. Today, three surgeons walked
All the way here—where two women bear their yoke—
Pulling, listening, feeding, charting. Here, read the next page:

One furniture store opened its doors to stranded
travelers & many others slept on floors in hotel lobbies.

Alice Kuhar and Joseph Brian's wedding didn't happen.
Doris DeBold sent her husband out with 5 gallons
of coffee and twenty sandwiches to the municipal light
plant where 33 men have been working non-stop 24 hours.
Business & Professional Women's Club cancelled
Mrs. Shepherd's talk on "You & Your Government."
Western Union has full time work for BOYS 16–18 *years*
of age, hourly rate. Apply in person. Mr. Mangus.
Dorsel's Restaurant on Euclid needs GIRLS-WOMEN,
Day or Night. Experience unnecessary. Salary, tips, meals
and uniforms. Apply 10:30 A.M. and 2:30 P.M.

Seven patients are vomiting; six have diarrhea.
Four complained of chest pain. They cannot call home.
Visitors cannot make it in. Alma and I
Don't know if the next shift will show up.
Alma's knee grows shiny and hot, twisted, this morning

On ice—if only she could rest. Lunch trays are cold.
At the beginning of my shift, the supervisor said
I'd have to carry all the trash to the elevators.
When I was down the hall getting Mr. Grobinsky
Off his bedpan, I heard a patient yell at Alma.
Ours is not the only town in trouble:

In Poza Rica, an eastern Mexico oil town, poisonous
refinery smog snuffed out the lives of fifteen villagers
while they slept; sixty people have been hospitalized.
Smoke from the refinery plant mixed
with heavy fog, and cold night air, held it there
like a plastic bag over the faces of people sleeping.

Rebecca Ann Needham Anderson

Born in Miami, Oklahoma, October 2, 1957, Rebecca Ann Needham Anderson knew at an early age that she wanted to become a nurse. Rebecca was reared in a home with five siblings; her parents, Doris and Bob Needham, taught their children to be mindful of the less fortunate. This environment and her natural love and caring for all living things helped guide her decision to become a caregiver; when her youngest child left for school, Rebecca began to pursue her dream of nursing. She spoke often and fondly of her favorite nursing instructor, Mignon Denyer. Like many healthcare professionals, Rebecca was concerned about the shortage of competent nurses, the long hours nurses work, and the lack of dedication some nurses may display because of burnout.

Nurses often bring home stories about odd patients, cranky colleagues, and wild workdays. Work in an extended-care facility for the elderly gave Rebecca plenty of stories. She appreciated the male nurses and had a good rapport with physicians. The mother of four children, Gabriel, Hilary, Rachael, and Britton, Rebecca was skilled in care-giving, communication, and organization. No doubt her years of setting limits and providing positive reinforcement for expected behaviors served her well in this small community of wrinkled grannies and grandpas. Some patients refused to communicate until they found someone to trust. Rebecca often told the story of a female patient who the staff believed was

Rebecca Needham Anderson, 1994. (Courtesy Doris Needham.)

mute because she never spoke. One day the elderly woman asked Rebecca if she knew a certain hymn. Surprised, Rebecca was happy to say, "I do know that hymn, because I'm a singer, too."

When Rebecca heard the shocking news of the bombed Alfred P. Murrah Federal Building in Oklahoma City, April 19, 1995, she and her husband, Fred, rushed to the scene. Rebecca entered the building and pulled two survivors from the rubble. She went back a third time and led another person to safety. In the process of attempting to save more lives, Rebecca sustained head trauma, and despite surgery, died from those injuries. Knowing Rebecca's commitment to organ donation, her family asked that her heart and kidneys be recovered for transplant. In May 2003 Rebecca Anderson received the America's Heroes of Freedom: Women Are Heroes Too award in Washington D.C. Rebecca loved humanity enough to give her best, give her all, and give her life.

CALL AND RESPONSE

Rebecca Anderson, nurse
who died from head injuries
after trying to rescue people
Oklahoma City bombing

So, this is the smell of trouble, the taste of blood.
Me, buried in rubble, trying to raise my left hand,
an answer, finally, to the teacher's question.
Over here, I want to say to the siren's scream,

the sound of men telling me: *stay back, get back.*
Your sewing machine's too far away, Mom,
and besides, there's no mending me now.
I grew tired of white ceilings, watching the game

and never running a stop sign. Courage blooms,
a clap of thunder in a dry forest, and maybe lightning's
the world's faint pulse, the point of life.
What have I done today, to make the world better?

Miss Simpson wrote on her blackboard, then turned
around, wheezing, facing us. In sixth grade,
it was call and response, me chewing M&Ms,
dreaming of marrying Donny Osmond.

But now, the medic's coffee breath above
me, his penlight checks my pupils. My head's
kicked in, a bruised soccer ball half-filled with grit.
So, this is the wind's roar, the hungry wolf's yellow grin.

I want to say, *Yes, I forgot myself, forgot my hardhat*
to these firemen who are lifting me,
to the men shouting:
crazy woman, woman without a brain.

BIRCH CANOE

for Lieutenant Dan Suttles

After supper, my daughter asked me,
Any bad stuff today?

I would like to answer *no*, but she's seen
the six o'clock news, yellow tape surrounding
the trailer's shell, the story of sisters playing with matches,
our fire captain, tired, begging parents to put lighters up,

install smoke alarms. She knows the child named Sara
came to my hospital. I am touched by her concern,
Will they make it, Mom? I try to tell her about the fireman,
young and sweaty and mustached, his scorched suit

kneeling beside our gurney, holding swollen sooty fingers
of a toddler he did not know, praying for this flower
he'd gone into the flames to gather. I try to tell her
about men who are gentle and strong, men who rise

without hesitation, become larger than themselves
and do not paint their faces with arrows
and do not thump their chests blue. I do not know
how they tell themselves not to be afraid,

how they let the black smoke swallow them over and over.
I just know tonight this fireman was a birch canoe;
he swam into the fire and pulled Sara back into this world
that is never easy.

Betty Jane Panchik

Acknowledging that women wear many hats in one lifetime, Betty Jane Panchik worked as a full-time emergency medical technician for seventeen years prior to her nursing education. As a nontraditional nursing student at Sharon General Hospital in Sharon, Pennsylvania, she continued to work her full-time job. Seeing such dedication to the healthcare field, her employer wanted to retain B.J. with his ambulance service. When she was offered a wage similar to that which she would receive in hospital nursing service, she continued to serve the EMS community for another seven years. Eventually she left the EMS and began working in three local steel mills as an occupational health nurse.

A member of the American Association of Occupational Health Nurses, B.J. is known as the "Sweetheart of the Melt Shop" to hundreds of employees at three Ohio steel mills. Involved with such a diverse socioeconomic population, B.J. believes it is a privilege to care for "well" people. Ergonomic related injuries and prolonged exposure to chemicals are ongoing issues for the personnel in the steel industry. As a team, the plant physician and B.J. monitor hearing conservation, foster education about common health problems such as hypertension and diabetes, and have recently implemented a smoking cessation wellness program.

The potential for explosions, burns, and multiple trauma is present in her field of nursing, and safety issues are stressed daily by management and by B.J.

B. J. Panchik, 1997. (Author's collection.)

Employees show up at her door with headaches and mangled limbs, sore throats and myocardial infarctions. Her skilled triage assessments and EMS background facilitate the care of those needing immediate attention. B.J. receives hugs and flowers and small gifts from people who have benefited from her sound nursing judgment. She thinks all nurses should receive "respect from administration and physicians because they work hand in hand with them." She is now the nurse manager of Forum Health's work-med unit. B.J. has no regrets in her career choice; "It fulfills a need for self-esteem and nurturing in me. Since I never had children, my patients are my kids. I like being a helper." Currently enrolled at Penn State to obtain her nursing degree, she proudly tells her husband and others she's obtaining additional education "because it opens more doors for all of us."

NOVEMBER 1963

B J. Panchik, nurse, occupational health

The girl I was sits on the kitchen floor
moves her father's rag undershirt back
and forth across her mother's nursing shoes.
Where mother's foot had been, I slide my hand,
feel how her weight has stretched the leather,
each sewn part grown to fit her toes,
some powder she sprinkled inside drifts
its dust into the air. I pull the silent tongue,
see how the laces have crossed themselves,
her heels suffer their slants. This close,
I cannot escape the layered smells of sweat.
I am eight years old, third grade,
and already I have learned how blood dries
a rusty brown, how it freckles her shoes,
stains her uniforms. Tuesday's my night
to shake the pale liquid and smooth it on;
halfway down each shoe the leather cracks,
a gray scar from so many missions.
With the rag's soft ribs I rub and rub and rub
until the white's like the satin sash
on my communion dress. In two weeks,
we'll wash the good dishes, polish silver,
hear a wishbone's snap after the turkey's carved.

In Dallas, our president will be shot,
and for days my parents will stare
at the TV set and each other,
newspapers will be saved.
A small boy will salute a flag-draped casket,
and my sister will have her turn shining
our mother's shoes—a ceremony
thanking her for every step of her life.

$\mathscr{T}$he mother of three daughters, Hortense Wood has slowly been climbing the professional nursing ladder for more than thirty-four years. This energetic woman has balanced several roles to reach her present job as director of nurses at an Ohio correctional facility. A full-time wife, mother, and employee, she is a 1999 Youngstown State University graduate with her BSN. A native of Ohio, she is one of the original six nurses hired at the local Trumbull County correctional facility. When asked about preparation to work with an inmate population, she responds, "We had three weeks of training sessions to learn rules and regulations, security issues, and self defense. [We learned that] sharps must be accounted for properly; otherwise there's a lockdown until they are found. We learned to shoot a gun and pistol. My husband was a hunter, so I already knew how to handle a shotgun. In fact, I did so well on the target range they called me *Rambette.*"

Hortense was very instrumental in setting up the medical unit. No doubt, her many years of experience as a staff nurse in an urgent-care facility, an occupational health nurse at a local steel mill, a hospital staff nurse in med-surg units, and a charge nurse provided a wealth of resources for organizing the prison's medical unit. She is truly a team member. Hortense is a returning adult student, and her nursing professors have noted her eagerness to assist fellow classmates with their own assignments.

Hortense Thomas, graduation, 1964, Choffin School of Practical Nursing. (Courtesy Hortense Wood.)

"Nursing is hard work. Even years ago when my husband and I were dating, my thighs ached at night. He bought me a heating pad for them so they wouldn't hurt so badly while we played cards with friends. The heating pad helped my legs some, but I still watched the clock; at twelve, we had to go. I was just too tired on my weekends to work."

Certified in Correctional Health Care Management and HIV counseling, Hortense reports, "When I toured the prison, it was empty and had an eerie feeling to it. My father encouraged me to work at the prison. At first, my mother was fearful about this job, but now she knows I'm safe. We [the nurses] don't need to know what crime put an inmate here; we are here for the medical care of patients. This is very interesting work, and I like what I do. We have a lot of chronic problems in this population: diabetes, hypertension, asthma, and psych disorders. There's a full-time psychiatrist on staff and psychologists." Hortense works very closely with her medical director and feels the nurse-physician relationships have definitely improved since she began nursing.

After ten years she left the correctional facility to teach nursing, and she's pleased with her career move. While she loves to express her creativity by sewing everything from wedding gowns to tailored suits, her hectic schedule has crowded out the pinking shears and bolts of satin for now. When asked if she would become a nurse again, she responds, "Yes, nurses can move around to other areas, but I love my work and cannot see myself in any other career."

AT THIRTEEN, I DECIDE TO BECOME A NURSE

Hortense Wood, director of nurses, Ohio prison

At thirteen, I had the legs of a colt and the breasts
of a sparrow. How to become as lovely as Lena Horne?
One July, I was sick—appendicitis—a doctor's pale hands
touched my belly. Say you were me, a girl with skin

the color of rubbed chestnuts, a kid who'd never slept
under sheets her Mama didn't wash.
Say no one but your Mama had ever seen you naked,
but right then your belly's so full of hurt

you were a paper doll on fire. The doctor's voice said,
"Lie still and flat; make your tummy soft."
His clumsy fingers stepped over tender regions
of your abdomen like he's a farmer setting fence posts.

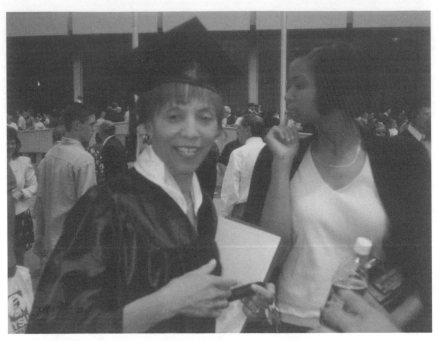

Hortense Wood and her daughter, Courtney, at Hortense's 1999 graudation, BSN, Youngstown State University. (Courtesy Hortense Wood.)

The hospital halls were backyards busy with women
in white shoes, starched caps and dresses sewn of snow.
Were they churches with their doors thrown open?
These women with pear hips and the faces of Mary

who moved small alcohol swabs and marched, not alone,
but in legions through morning pills, lunch trays,
sleepy flashlight nights. Mama said *angels of mercy;*
Daddy said *pride.* I chose this life.

In nursing, I learned snowflakes are born in old men's socks.
For extra pudding, grannies trade stories: *Every spring in my village*
we laced flowers around the cows' necks, and Mama made for me
a velvet vest and skirt that swirled a wide circle while I danced with Papa.

They will tell you such things,
die in your arms, and for days
your hair smells like smoke.

WARBLERS

When we wrestle soft old people
into their beds, clawing and shriveled,
I can't help thinking freedom is instinct
and falling is no worse
than flying without wings.

In wheelchairs, they become reels
of silent movies, gray and terribly sad,
dressed in flapping arms
and pale blue gowns.

Hasn't the sky already tumbled?
Their ribs are paper kites
lonely for sunset
and lunging in short bursts
from their chests.

What can I do but catch this string,
Fasten it to our steel, keep them
From blowing into thickets
Or over the edge of boulders?

I find it impossible not to imagine
them before—pink and round and barefoot—
racing each other in cool spring air,
where, suddenly, their cries become warblers
who can't stop calling for help
before the cat creeps back
grinning, waving his midnight tail.

Jane Ball

*A*n Ohio native and mother of seven children, Jane Ball has forty years of nursing service to her credit. She and her siblings are the first generation of their family to obtain professional educations, and Jane especially admired her older sister, a registered nurse. When Jane was a little girl, her dolls were always *sick* and sometimes in the hospital, so she had to care for them until they were better. When asked about nurses training, she remembers her first day was one of the best: "I was thrilled to be there." She is a diploma graduate and board certified in nursing administration.

Able to function well in many nursing areas, Jane has worked in the operating room, obstetrics, pediatrics, med-surg areas, emergency room, and with the code team. She credits one of her nursing instructors, Winifred Bassert, for instilling a love for disciplined nursing techniques during training. As a staff leader, she encouraged other team members to participate in critical situations and to continue their education for personal growth. While working general duty in emergency, Jane was asked to assume an administrative role when her supervisor took a pregnancy leave; the transition from general duty to supervision was so successful that eventually she became a supervisor until retirement. Jane notes, "Growth occurs in many ways when we share our knowledge; wages and benefits are only a small part of a nurse's benefits."

One aspect of nursing Jane has seen change over the years is the relationship

Jane Ball, 1998. (Author's collection.)

between doctors and nurses. Doctors are no longer "kings," and a nurse's knowledge is recognized as a valuable asset to the healthcare team. Still, she believes, "many people do not know the abilities and functions of nurses." She admits this is a generational opinion, but "when nurses removed their caps and uniforms, the public lost the ability to differentiate the levels of staff members caring for their loved ones." Jane is sure she would become a nurse again. "My career enhanced my self-esteem; my husband and children were proud of me." She admits, "I feel a sadness concerning nursing and medical care due to the political influences today. Nurses don't get credit for their efforts, which results in frustration." Her professional passion is "to try and improve patient care—empathy is the key."

WHAT NURSES DO: THE MARRIAGE OF SUFFERING AND HEALING

Jane Ball, retired nursing supervisor

Compared to the day I had to sit with a mother
Ask for her daughter's three-year-old kidneys,
Eyes, liver, and heart because a drunken
Teenager had killed her brain
Compared to the afternoon I told a black man
His son was shot while jogging
Compared to the night I was paged to ER
To help sedate a seven-year-old girl
Before they sewed her crotch
Being here with this schoolteacher holding
Her husband's hand, begging him to live
Is better.

The rhythm of a heart repeats itself like vows
In a chapel full of light, but we are gathered
Here because this man's heart choked after forty years
Medics shocked him, brought him back
Then, a cardiologist with his pacemaker, a respirator
We have stolen these minutes
But our bag has no more tricks, no more drugs
Or gizmos, and now, something as old as love
Must be the pencil that helps the heart write
Its good-byes across our screen.

I will never forget the wife's brown hair
And her tan corduroy blazer, how her face looked
When she asked for her husband's baptism
We couldn't reach a priest. It happens.
They all looked at me: the nursing supervisor.
I said I could.
In the presence of this company
Who gives this man to the next world?
The paper cup was blue, I asked a blessing
For the tap water and did it, water fell
Soft as a kiss to his forehead.

And so I kept the devil far away
And let the wife cry into my shoulder
For a long time after
For a long time after.

June Elizabeth Connolly

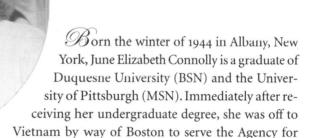

$\mathcal{B}$orn the winter of 1944 in Albany, New York, June Elizabeth Connolly is a graduate of Duquesne University (BSN) and the University of Pittsburgh (MSN). Immediately after receiving her undergraduate degree, she was off to Vietnam by way of Boston to serve the Agency for International Development; she had been trained to care for people with tropical diseases. The plans changed; she did not go to Saigon. Instead she worked with Vietnamese patients at Massachusetts General for the next twelve months. Many of the patients were small children and women whose injuries included severe burns, amputations, and multiple traumas. Burned out after a year, June returned to Pittsburgh. The war's shadow followed her. She remembers that a ten o'clock curfew was maintained due to protest riots over Vietnam.

In Pittsburgh, June was excited about working with two pioneer heart surgeons who implemented the mammary artery transplant for cardiac surgery. She clearly remembers losing many of the early cardiac patients, and some died very slowly in reverse isolation. In nursing and life June reports, "There are too many battles and not enough time." Her next position was in a surgical intensive care unit, where she performed hemodialysis: "It was a mathematical equation you could solve every day. Patients got well, at least for a while."

In the late 1960s she married and moved to a smaller town, where she became a diploma school instructor. In 1970 she realized more education was an

June Elizabeth Connolly, 1997. (Courtesy June Connolly.)

investment in her future. "I loved all the anatomy and physiology classes. Four days a week I commuted to Pittsburgh. Many of my classes were with the pre-med students." Upon completing her master's degree, June had several job offers, but her husband was an established businessman and deeply rooted in his community, so she looked for a job locally. A cardiologist asked June to help him design and manage a cardiac-rehab facility.

It was challenging work, and she worked nearly sixty hours a week. While working at that facility, she had two miscarriages; then, at age thirty-six, a successful pregnancy. "I thought I'd be home a few weeks with Patrick (my son) and go back to work. After four weeks, I called to say I needed more time off. At the end of that stretch, I knew I didn't want to go back to work. They gave me an extended leave of absence, but I ended up handing in my resignation. Throughout my son's toddler years, I worked maybe one day every other week; I could talk to adults and keep my hand in medicine."

From 1988 to 1989, June went back to a clinical-instructor teaching position at a regional college, but she was still looking for a schedule that corresponded with her family's needs. A school nurse job became available, and she had no trouble securing the position.

As a member of the social justice organization Witness for Peace, June traveled to Nicaragua in the summer of 1990 with other concerned health caregivers. In Nicaragua's isolated and impoverished areas, she saw huge waste incinerators being built along the Atlantic coast. An active environmentalist, June realizes improper handling of toxic substances potentially endangers people's lives. She viewed a proposed waste incinerator for East Liverpool as a threat to the environment and community, so she lifted her voice in protest. She was no longer "killing myself to give good nursing care" and saw that she had a pivotal position in the community to be an advocate for children.

A former member of the intra-aortic balloon pump team, June understands the thin line separating life and death and the way silence gives consent. She is committed to speaking her mind and keeping the public informed. "Because I've done so many different things with nursing, I'd definitely become a nurse again."

SCHOOL NURSE

June Connolly, nurse, environmental activist

My students are not dairy cattle, I don't say
hey this, hey that. Strep rides the throat
with a mean whip, unchecked,
it slides to the heart, the kidneys.

On soft bellies of kindergartners, I read
braille vesicles of chicken pox.

My fingers sort through scalps, spring,
winter, fall, find quilting stitches of lice,
pink coins of ringworm. A clinician, I make
students bend over, bend over, a spine aslant
is a train derailed, it can cripple, it breathes
under lace bras and football jerseys.

Their bodies are sexual, a flask of holy water,
I tell teens there's no neutral state of lying,
herpes blooms forever, green penile discharge
doesn't come from toilet seats, a missed period's
not a grammar problem. Sometimes, we hurt each other
without meaning to—all of us.

Family sacredness means children are not ashtrays
or wheat to be crushed, a hand-shaped bruise
shows fungus breeding a cesspool. The art of brewing
chamomile tea does little to warm Iris,
a nine-year-old who staggers from her bus
like the last man to leave the ring.

Certain screams bring my first assignment back: 1968
Mass. General, women, children maimed in Vietnam.
Wards full of pain in another tongue. They came,
tags pinned to their dressings, names I could not
pronounce or now remember. Asian dolls without legs,
charred flesh, blind boys touching me, touching me.

When the EPA gave the OK to build an incinerator 1100 feet
from my school's door, I mailed protest letters
to the board, was arrested in D.C., fought to stop future
mutant strains. Now, I collect emergency care sheets,
watch for eating disorders, show the films on puberty,
screen for vision, screen for vision.

$\mathscr{A}$ 1969 graduate of the Sisters of Charity School of Nursing in Kansas City, Kansas, Helen Krier remembers her first excitement over wearing a student uniform and cap. To earn the title of registered nurse, she fought her test fears; she has never been proficient at examinations. In fact, three months before she graduated from training, her director called her into the office to say that she didn't expect Helen to be successful at state board examinations. The director went on to explain, "It's not because you lack knowledge, you just can't take tests." Helen realized the director was right, but it was one of the most painful moments in her nursing life. Maybe the meeting was a catalyst to defeat test anxiety, because Helen passed her boards the first time.

The first person in her family to obtain a professional education, Helen has worked with several extraordinary colleagues over the years. Her long-time friend and hospice mentor, Anna French, "was the first nurse that I met and truly admired." Helen admits that until she went into hospice nursing, she had tried to figure out "what I could do to get out of nursing and make enough money to support my kids as a single parent." And while she thought about furthering her nursing education over the years, she was disappointed to find most of her diploma credits would not transfer. Even with fifteen years of experience, she'd have to invest almost as much time in a baccalaureate degree as any other freshman.

Helen Krier, 1998. (Author's collection.)

Like most nurses, she has felt the displaced anger of physicians. Once, while working surgery, a physician told her "if I don't get a pacemaker in my patient, she [the patient] will die and it will be your [Helen's] fault." The physician shouted all of this in front of the patient's family and the entire ICU staff. Other physicians were outraged by such behavior and went to administration; the cardiologist had to call her to his office to apologize. Helen handed in her resignation anyway, but today, she believes, the doctor/nurse relationships are much more cohesive, especially in hospice.

It's impossible to escape death while performing bedside nursing. When she was hired to work in a nursing home, her supervisor told her "to expect approximately three deaths on her shift." Helen's goal was to make sure that nobody died until her shift was finished, and she convinced herself it was her *special care* holding death at bay. Now, she believes it was her own fear of dying, and reports, "People have an intuitive sense of who is comfortable being present at the time of their death." They respond accordingly. Thirteen years after she passed her state boards, Helen could no longer sidestep the emotional landmine of death when she cared for a young man who had lung cancer in 1982. Also that year, she attended her first death and dying workshop where "I released a lot of tears and fears of dying. I decided to go into hospice. I thought if I could teach people how to die, maybe they could teach me how to live."

Her greatest joy in nursing was obtaining hospice certification in 1997. It was the first test Helen had taken since state boards in 1969, and passing it "gave me a great deal of self confidence." She also comments, "it's sad to think what kind of fears we allow ourselves to be crippled by." In 1999 she took a leap of faith and opened her Oregon home to hospice patients. One-hundred-three people have chosen Helen's hospice as their final spot to anchor down: "There was a time in my life that I felt I wanted to do something that would make me famous, and I used to stress about this a great deal. It occurred to me, I had already accomplished this by raising two beautiful children who have turned into wonderful adults that contribute a great deal to society." She's not sure if she would be a nurse again but she probably would not, because "nursing is going away from patient care and becoming more administrative and computerized. A nurse's responsibility is not reflected in her salary."

CHRISTMAS IS ANOTHER MOON

Helen Krier, hospice nurse

The nurse, Helen, pulls into the driveway.
She brings medicine, a poultice to draw
Water from a grandfather's lungs. Today
He asks for truth, close to the prairie, eyes raw
From its dust. *Can you get me through Christmas?*
She opens her leather pouch, mixes magic vials.
Christmas is another moon. Her answer's frost.
Filled syringes build a raft for ten more miles.
He clings to a branch in this river's flood.
He coughs, a wolf eating carrion chokes.
She listens: breath sounds, heart sounds, a drum's blood.
Messages painted on ancient faces, smoke,
Stories of mountain passes, wood burning,
And winter trees and blue sky opening.

Darrell Grace

Being denied acceptance into three schools of nursing did not discourage Dr. Darrell Grace. Nursing was one important step on the career ladder for this dynamic Youngstown, Ohio, woman. After a visit with her high school guidance counselor, she went home and told her grandmother, "He wanted to know when I was getting married." Darrell's grandmother responded, "Over my dead body." Reared by a family who "loved to help others," Darrell learned by example to be compassionate and nurturing. "My mother was a nurse's aide, and my grandmother had her beauty shop on the back of our house. She [grandmother] was always doing free hair."

In 1968 Darrell's stepfather went knocking on university doors after she'd received rejection letters. "Please tell me why my stepdaughter can't be a student here. Show me where she doesn't meet the requirements." When her transcripts were examined, administrators could not find any deficiencies. They apologized, and Darrell was admitted the next term to Youngstown State University, where she completed an associate degree in nursing in 1975 and a bachelor's degree in health sciences in 1987. These degrees laid the groundwork for her studies at Michigan State University College of Osteopathic Medicine, where she graduated in 1992.

Prior to becoming a physician, Darrell worked as a staff nurse, a head nurse, a supervisor, and a private-duty and per-diem nurse in Ohio and Michigan emer-

Darrell Grace, 1998. (Author's collection.)

gency rooms. "As a nurse and, later, as a physician, I was angered when any patient was mistreated because they didn't have money. I promised myself all patients under my care would be treated with respect no matter what." As a woman of color she admits she had "extra battles to fight" while pursuing her educational goals. And "those battles take your energy away from your studies. There are lots of hoops and hurdles. You have to keep going."

She recalls one of her medical professors telling the residents, "Take your own blood pressures; the nurses don't know how to take blood pressures." Darrell's hand flew up immediately, and her professor's face turned crimson. "First, don't believe that. Since I've been in med school, I've been teaching other students how to take blood pressures. No one has taught us. It's like we were supposed to already know it. Second, if you treat a nurse like she's stupid, she'll be stupid all night long with phone calls to you. If you treat her like she's smart, she'll be smart." The professor apologized; he had forgotten he had nurses in his classroom.

Committed to her faith and community, Darrell graduated in Michigan and returned to Youngstown, Ohio, to practice medicine in the inner-city clinic Grace Place. There are weeks when she is so busy that "there's no time to cry, and I think crying cleanses the soul." She believes that nurses need more camaraderie and less underhanded behaviors, "because it diminishes what we can accomplish." Darrell would become a nurse again "in a New York minute. I love the time one gets to spend with the patient as a nurse, but students are not taught, or should I say it is not focused on as much in medical school." Darrell was the recipient of the Richard L. Alper Award for Community Service when she graduated from Michigan State University College of Osteopathic Medicine.

WHEN I TELL MY MOTHER I WANT TO BE A DOCTOR

Dr. Darrell Grace, former ER nurse

Mother is in the Ohio cellar
where her brown hands
cannot quit throwing clothes.
Moving in the air, socks
with no mates, she separates
parts of the mass.

My voice belongs to a girl
dressed in anklets and buckled shoes.
A girl who remembers quiet rows

of cookies, the pale smiles
of gingerbread men kept
inside the baker's case.

I want to be a doctor,
I've applied to med school.
What do you think?
Her fingers knead thick towels
like they are bread dough.
She checks the pockets

Of muddy jeans, soaks a bloody
shirt. The First Lady of gentle loads,
stray dimes, handfuls
of gray dryer lint. She knows
a dream blessed becomes flesh.
I am grown, a nurse, twenty-eight,

And daughters in Zaire
find their way using stars for a compass.
What moon decides
the hungry faces of tent people,
the dying stares of mothers
who cannot hush their crying bundles?

She cannot geld the lions
circling ahead. She nods
for me to lift the basket's weight.
Her ancient eyes say,
Child, come along with me,
and bring those wooden pins.

Judy Waid

$\mathcal{J}$n the forty-plus years since Judy Waid graduated from Trumbull Memorial Hospital School of Nursing in Warren, Ohio, she has witnessed many changes in healthcare. Originally hired as a staff nurse on a twenty-four-bed unit in 1959 for $1.35 an hour, she now recalls having nightmares after shifts when she "had rotating tourniquets all the way down the hall, no aid to help, and was supposed to be passing medications. There wasn't even time to call the supervisor and cry on the phone." When she and her husband looked at their first baby, she thought, "It would be wonderful to just keep having babies." After this baby, Judy's family physician asked her to work part-time in his doctor's office, and her wages paid for the entire cost of the delivery.

Destined to be a mother, Judy had four babies in five years. She accepted a part-time afternoon charge-nurse position at a nearby rehab hospital when her youngest child was two. The baby cried at the door when she left; none of the kids wanted Dad to wash their hair; supper leftovers and dishes were waiting for her when Judy opened the door at midnight. Her husband really didn't want her to work. So after eight months she resigned, and, for a time, she didn't miss all the confusion and stress of nursing. Already, a psych patient had thrown a bedpan full of urine on her, and she'd cared for a young ballet dancer with severe brain stem injury, which left her in a fetal position. Balancing a family and a career is tough. Judy's own mother was a nurse, and she remembers, "I hated it when she worked."

Judy Waid, 1997. (Author's collection.)

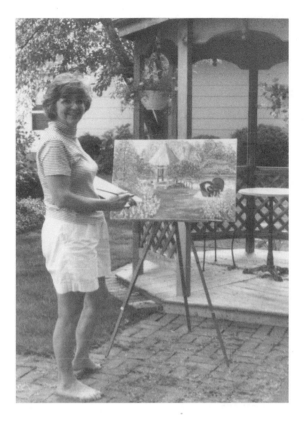

In 1970 she received a phone call from a nurse friend who worked at the rehab hospital: "We need a part-time midnight nurse. Will you try it?" It was close to home, and she was ready. Finally, Judy accrued enough seniority to earn paid vacation. "I was delighted. We packed and went camping at the lake." She worked ten years of night turn, then filled a day-turn staff nurse position. "It was mostly spinal cord injuries, young people who were very challenging. Cord injuries sap your strength. Later, it was drug abuse mixed with cord injuries. Sometimes, parental support wasn't there, and my patients didn't want to accept their disabilities." It takes time for any nurse to learn that nurse goals and patient goals are on different timetables.

"I was the middle child in my family and born with a crayon in my hand," Judy responds when asked about her love for painting. "Before I was old enough to go to school, I'd walk down the street, and the nuns would let me in the schoolhouse. I'd be very quiet and draw pictures of them. They liked having me around." Judy started painting while in high school, and between family and job responsibilities she managed to attend art classes at the Butler Art Institute Museum in Youngstown, Kent State University, and the Cleveland Institute of Art. Some of her paintings are part of the permanent collection at Hillside Rehabilitation

Hospital, and she was chosen to design the commemorative medallions for the Ohio Nurses Association from 1990 to 1995 and in 1997. Each medallion celebrates a different historical nurse leader or event. Having finished her nursing career in the tuberculosis clinic, an outpatient clinic, and in employee health programs, Judy enjoys gardening, landscape, nature, impressionist-realist painting, and being a grandmother. Looking back on her career choice, "I think I'd become a nurse again, but I'd have my BSN and masters, or at least a BFA."

PENTIMENTO

Judy Waid, artist, retired nurse, spinal-cord rehab

Another morning at my canvas—my day off,
no wheelchairs or spoons fastened to spasmed hands.
I'm expecting the soft repetition of shoots
and blossoms, shadows and changing bodies of light.

I stand close to the easel and hold my brush,
my breath. It's a gamble to paint faces,
gasping jaws of tulips, lazy yawns of daisies,
necks blooming white stems.

After twenty-two years,
I make bold sweeping gestures
as if I've earned the right to free
what can be developed in this space.

A village where the day is bright and sunny,
a raked terrace around the blue cafe,
green vines erase the building's torn spine
and cradle clusters of pink buds.

Look, there, leading up the hillside, a girl
with small braids, a boy in overalls,
a mother in her cotton dress.
To increase strength, I make them hold hands.

Intimacy creates motion, a desire to climb,
to use their legs, to run

and not be contained. Inside the café
voices flutter, an iridescent dance

of cups and bowls and hunger,
a sort of happiness, sliced thick
and warm as fresh bread, a room
where women ladle steamy soup

for fishermen in gray woolen caps
and the talk is all salt and noodles,
the efforts of daily life.
The woman brings my food, my spoon,

and for a while, I forget
everything but the broth
and the music of these voices.

Lynda Arnold

*B*orn in Pennsylvania, Lynda Arnold always knew she wanted a career in the medical field. "I wanted to be a doctor or a singer, but I had to look at things practically, so I became a nurse by default. I received an ROTC nursing scholarship, and after the first tough year, I really loved nursing." She is one of five daughters, and her family is full of helpers. Her mother and sister are teachers, and one sister is in the Peace Corps.

A BSN graduate of York College of Pennsylvania, her best experience in training was witnessing the delivery of a baby. She especially remembers two fellow students from training: "a man who is now a missionary nurse traveling everywhere and a woman who became a midwife." She has many positive thoughts about nursing and nursing training: "I think it's great to travel with your family while doing nursing. My college friend who is now a midwife didn't even choose nursing until her sophomore year at college. She's doing great."

Lynda believes her mother was an important mentor, and she's thankful to be living close to her parents now. Lynda was working less than a year when she received a needle stick from one of her patients who was in full-blown, end-stage AIDS. "I remember when I had to go in for the second test results. The secretary did not look happy, and she was a person who always smiled. I was alone when they told me I was HIV positive. I called my best friend, a law student, and wanted to get out of the office."

Lynda Arnold, 1997. (Courtesy Lynda Arnold.)

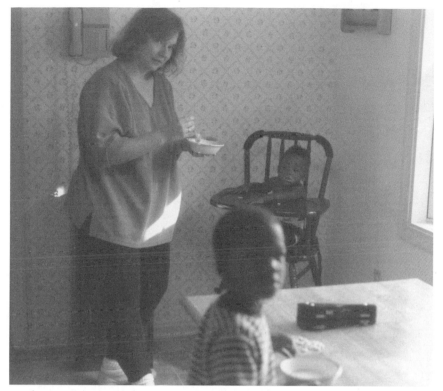

Lynda, David, and Ashley Arnold, 1997. (Author's collection.)

As her world came apart, she looked for things to hold on to. She was dating Tony Arnold. Would he still want to date her knowing she was ill? "I'd always wanted a family and marriage. As it turned out, Tony stayed with me and we married. I was Catholic and worried about the rules of the church. I didn't know if I could get married with HIV in my church. The priest was very open-minded and supportive. My husband has been wonderful; we value our relationship and are very close."

Lynda and her husband moved near Philadelphia and after adopting two children had a child of their own. All of the children are healthy, and each has added joy to the Arnold home. David is seven years old, Ashley's five, and Michael's three. A spokesperson for the National Conference of Healthcare Workers' Safety, Lynda completed her MBA in May 2002, currently works full time, and travels around the country to educate all age groups concerning HIV.

She advises new nurses: "Listen to your patients; know what you are doing; if you don't know what you're doing, get help; don't be afraid to bend the rules a little when it comes to patients and their families." She believes a nurse earns respect as she or he travels through the ranks. When asked about anger she replies, "Learn to forgive early, and move past your anger because it gets you nowhere." As to her own health on a daily basis: "I laugh a lot, cry a lot, take one day at a time, don't plan too far ahead, and I allow myself to dream." Her health is holding steady; with only one recent hospitalization Lynda continues to focus on the future, where she plans to keep stepping up to the plate and swinging hard.

BEGIN AGAIN

for Lynda Arnold, nurse, HIV positive

They meet, bent over to drink from one stream,
their faces close as apples on a branch,
and mountain water so cold their teeth ache.

Tenderness, his forehead's purple mark is gone,
some granny's hand has patted it back to earth.
A nurse, her patient, they are not strangers.

She blushes from this closeness, the bodice
of her gauzy dress touches each breast.
Opacity, the origin of forms, his new body,

so tan and full, cotton shirt blown open
in a breeze. *Warm day,* she says, smoothing
her hair and staring at the meadow

holding its bouquet of wildflowers like a bride.
He nods, kneels, jeans faded, pockets walletless.
Smell the pine? He asks. She shuts her eyes,

breathes the sap's blue jazz.
Every day thin needles die and drop,
a symbol to begin again, to find an answer.

His fingers lift her hand.
Is this where my needle caught your glove?
She nods, sits down.

Do you remember the snow, she says,
how it fell on your face softer than sugar
then melted like tears?

Yes, yes, he answers. All around them movement,
organza skirts of poppies flushed and twirling
lacy parasols—a dance, a waltz.

Silence, a pause before the starting line.
What do you miss? They ask each other,
speaking slowly, knowing it was an accident,

Meeting there, here, and the question's a wound,
a drop of blood no longer visible.
Their words scatter across the fields,

so small we cannot see them.
They float through the air saying *nothing*
nothing, singing forgiveness.

Part 7

There is this edge where shadows
and bones of some of us walk backwards.

Joy Harjo, "Call It Fear"

The Sisters of St. Joseph's Hospitallers

In the 1600s a voyage across the Atlantic ocean
meant more than two months of wind, waves, hardship, and a bit of luck. The
newly formed French colony of Montreal was in desperate need of nursing
personnel. Since it was a coastal colony, ships and sailors arrived there with
typhus and blankets, smallpox and food. The native Iroquois were a constant
source of danger for the colonists. At great risk of life and safety, in 1659 three
Sisters of St. Joseph's Hospitallers sailed from France with Jeanne Mance, a
Catholic lay nurse, to care for the diverse population of Montreal's inhabitants.

On their arrival, they found their quarters had more than two hundred holes
in it, where wind and snow entered constantly. Living in the settlement's most
decrepit buildings, the first work each morning was to shovel and sweep away
the snow. Food was scarce, and the provisions available were barely edible. The
church appropriated resources for medications and instruments for the hospital, Hotel Dieu. Hotel Dieu was established in 1642 by Jeanne Mance to serve
the sick and impoverished population of Montreal. The missionary pioneers
of St. Joseph's Hospitallers converted the natives, bandaged the explorers, and
cared tirelessly for each other. The sisters prevailed despite language barriers,
lack of supplies, and harsh winters in poor housing. Faith was the fire that sustained them winter upon winter.

The settlement's newly built hospital was of wood construction, approximately
sixty feet by twenty-four feet. It contained a kitchen; a room for the hospital's
director, Jeanne Mance; one room for servants; and two rooms for the sick. A
small chapel and stable were built nearby, which were eventually furnished with
lamps and tables, chairs and livestock—all of which would arrive on summer

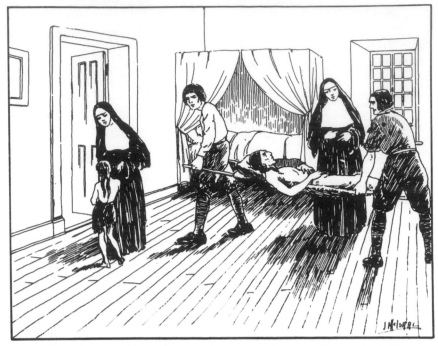

Patients' Ward of Hotel Dieu of Montreal, *seventeenth-century drawing by J. McIsaac.* *(Courtesy Religieuses Hospitalierès de St. Joseph, Montréal.)*

ships. In summer 1651 two hundred Iroquois attacked the hospital almost every day. The colonist were urged to move into Fort Ville Marie during this conflict. Thirty colonists perished, and Jeanne Mance requested that hospital funds be dispensed to French troops to protect the fort and hospital. One hundred men arrived to save the colony and ensure its survival. The Sisters of St. Joseph's Hospitallers lived through the 1662 earthquake (which they reported lasted for months), Iroquois wars, disease, and bone-chilling winters. Nearly 350 years later they remain as caregivers and spiritual leaders throughout the world.

INTERVIEW WITH SISTER DENIS OF ST. JOSEPH'S HOSPITALLERS COLONY OF MONTREAL, NEW FRANCE, 1694

Three months after the new hospital burnt down

—Your family is in France?
—That is true.
—How many novices started with you?
—Twenty.

—How many remain?
—Five.
—The rest?
—Took husbands in the Colony
—I have heard stories of trappers with frozen feet and scalped men crawling to the fort.
—That is true.
—And women found dead from childbirth in their cabins.
—Yes.
—And this is where you sleep?
—Yes.
—Isn't this the cellar of the granary?
—It is.
—But sister, the partitions are rotting, and here, see the wind pushes snow from all sides, surely the rain—
—We sleep back to back.
—But a good gust could take this ceiling. And the roof being so close to the floor—
—We pack the cracks with rags and straw.
—Sister, the brown loaf on the table? How are you able to slice frozen bread?
—We thaw it on the hearth.
—Is it true there was a fire?
—Yes.
—And your patients?
—Most of them jumped through the windows.
—And the sisters?
—They ran into the hospital garden.
—But it was winter and night.
—Yes.
—And was there ice? Wind?
—Yes.
—And did they have time to dress?
—They were in night garments.
—Shoes?
—No.
—Stockings?
—No.
—Your patients?
—Those who lived were taken into the seminary.
—The sisters?

—Were given hospitality by the Sisters of the Congregation.
—The habit you are boiling?
—It was Sister Dominic's.
—The habit on the table cut in squares?
—Was Sister Helene's.
—The habits that are draped and drying?
—Sister Anne, Sister Catherine, Sister Marie, Mother de Brésoles.
—They are bathing?
—They are dead.
—From the fire?
—From the sickness that starts with a blush and a fever, the purple rash that turns to pus.
—And you?
—I bled them, here, at the temple.
—And the priest?
—Confessed the dying.
—But I heard the supply ship also brought typhus?
—That is true.
—And the bodies of the dead were in piles?
—That is true.
—And the sisters fell ill in great numbers?
—That is true.
—And then?
—We accepted the offer of service from several good widows.
—Sister, those flea bites on your hands? Will you be going home?
—Soon, I will be going home.

Kate Cumming

*N*ever formally trained to become a nurse, Kate Cumming served tirelessly at the bedside of countless Confederate soldiers during the Civil War. A native of Scotland, she lived in Canada before her family moved to Alabama. It was here her father's employment as a clerk in banks and insurance companies created a solid foothold in middle-class society. Kate's decision to trade the security of her father's home for the difficult labor of nursing wounded soldiers was a source of great discord. After all, she was a *lady*, and nursing was not considered a proper job for women.

Ignorant of the life she was entering, Kate left Mobile with approximately forty other women to care for the soldiers arriving from the bloody battle of Shiloh. Many of her companions found the witnessing of war horrors was beyond bearing and returned home. True to her calling, Kate stayed and was enlisted as a hospital supervisor in 1862. New legislation allowed women to be employed by the Confederate medical department. Overcrowding and poor sanitation often caused illness among the caregivers and the soldiers. Work schedules were dictated by the push and pull of battles, supplies, and patient needs, not clocks.

Kate's legacy to the world is the journal she kept faithfully during her three years of dedicated service. In plain language, she transports her readers to another time and place: drained caregivers, agonizing moments of suffering, wagons stacked

Kate Cumming, ca. 1865, reproduced from the frontispiece of her Gleanings from Southland. *(Courtesy Library of Congress.)*

with bodies, blood running on floors like water. Almost ninety years after her death, Kate's naked grave was found and marked through the efforts of an admirer and historian, Art Green. In an impressive ceremony, which included a Confederate honor guard, retired nurses in their whites, and bagpipers, a white marble headstone graced a deserving humanitarian.

WAIT FOR MORNING: FROM KATE CUMMING'S JOURNAL

Confederate nurse, Civil War, 1862

APRIL 7
Arrived Okolona, Mississippi, with some ladies from Natchez and Mr. Skates who is on his way to bring back the remains of his son. Steady rain, no hotels, loss of sleep. We smelled them first, like spoiled crock sausage, those railroad cars filled with wounded passing through. Men, bleeding and moaning and mangled shadows through the slats.

APRIL 10
A carriage ride with Reverend Clute to Mrs. Henderson's. Her sister is a pianist. They are of Scotch descent. Both their husbands are in the army. She is using sweet potatoes instead of coffee until the war's end.

APRIL 11
Arrived Corinth, Mississippi. Raining washtubs. Water and mud, wagons stuck in slop. Yellow flags on hotels, taken for hospitals. Mrs. Ogden tried to prepare me, entering in the wards, lying on the floor, men like half-butchered steers, so close, to walk was to step on them. We passed cold biscuits and coffee. There are no plates. To wash and dress their wounds, we kneel in blood and water. After the first two hours, we don't notice our petticoats' red starch. An old man groans, his leg lost, a fine-looking man coughs, shot through his lungs, every drink of water bubbles out. This fog of urine and sweat baptizes the dying. What I saw there: men crowded in the hall, the gallery, small rooms, hands reaching up, and the air, stale and stopped. There is no order to war.

APRIL 13
Dr. Brown told me this morning his young wife, Emma, is alone on their plantation with more than a hundred Negroes, the only white man, his overseer. A satin lady came today with her parents in search of her husband, a colonel. Her mother presented me with several sperm candles.

APRIL 14

A number of bunks arrived today, and so some of the filth can be removed from this floor. Dr. Regan told me he thought a Federalist was in a bunk downstairs; if so, our men needed it. I asked another nurse; she would not take me to the Federalist. After a bit, I found him: a boy with blue eyes from Illinois shot through the jaw, crying for his mother, unable to drink. I left him to his blanket and bunk.

APRIL 17

Going my rounds as usual this morning washing the faces of men, I was half finished with one, when I saw he was dead. There is no end to it. Robert and William are two soldiers I cared for closely. When I asked the surgeon, he said they would not live another day. I went to them, thinking of my brother, David, somewhere fighting our enemy. I wrote their mothers, read Isaiah: *No lions will be there; no fierce animals will pass that way. Those whom the Lord has rescued will travel home by that road.*

APRIL 19

Received a letter from Mrs. Lucy Haughton and a box filled with eggs, crackers, fresh butter, and pickles, which the men relish. She is such a Christian woman. When the men first arrive, they eat just like pups suck, but in a few days, wounds flare, appetites leave them.

APRIL 23

A young man who I have been attending is to have his arm cut off. Daniel knows that he will die; all who have limbs amputated here have died. None of the prisoners have died yet. Our men do not seem to stand half so much as the Yanks. Dr. Hereford thinks our men will not endure camp life.

APRIL 24

When there is an amputation, I keep far away from the stairs' landing. Today, I had to pass that place. A warm stream of blood ran from the table to a washtub, over its edge, a motionless thing: a hand, unfastened like a woman's brooch, put down like a man's hat. A boy's opened fist.

APRIL 29

As we have no chaplain, we have no service. I read the Bible. There are no unbelievers, Baptists, Methodists, Presbyterians, or Roman Catholics. One hundred arrived last night on their way to another hospital. We fed those who would eat. I do not feel well. Other ladies are ill and doctors. I haven't the strength to write letters or coax broth tonight.

May 6

Mr. Jones, an eighteen-year-old, is dead. His leg was amputated. Mrs. Henderson sat with him all night. She wants a coffin for him, by God. In the beginning, I thought it awful to have men buried without them, but the living suffer so, that I pay little heed to those things. These men need no flaming ships or coffins to sail them into the land of glory. My first month is finished, and I try to believe Isaiah: *The desert will rejoice, and flowers will bloom in the wastelands.*

Jane Stuart Woolsey

On February 7, 1830, Jane Stuart Woolsey was born on a ship headed to New York. Her family then went to live in England with her father's parents for two years of her early life; then they returned to the United States and settled in Boston, where her father became a successful busi-nessman. When Jane was ten years old, her father drowned when the Long Island steamer *Lexington* sank. Mrs. Woolsey moved her nine children to New York near their well-to-do relatives. Jane and her sisters were educated at Rutgers's Female Institute. Mrs. Woolsey hated slavery, and Jane described herself and her brothers and sisters as "born abolitionists."

When the Civil War broke out, Jane was called to work in Alexandria, Virginia, at the Fairfax Seminary Hospital. Then in 1865 she became dietary and nursing supervisor for over two hundred wounded and ailing men housed in buildings that had been a divinity school. Some of the doctors resented Jane's presence and raised a fuss, but those were quickly replaced by order of the hospital board. Every man's name, diagnosis, and diet were written daily and the response to their nutrition and care recorded. Each patient had his own bottle labeled with his name; these were washed, dried, refilled, and corked daily. Food was delivered in wagons—which the patients called their "vittles trains"—with "buttoned doors on each side." Once it arrived, the food was guarded and trays

Jane Stuart Woolsey, ca. 1872. (Courtesy A. C. Long Health Science Library, Columbia University, New York.)

passed through open windows. Jane made daily rounds collecting criticisms and restructuring diets.

The majority of Jane's nurses were wives, sisters, and friends of soldiers. They often came to find family and stayed to serve. Some spoke German or French and were utilized as translators. These nurses (paid and unpaid) suffered dysentery, smallpox, and depression month after month. Tirelessly, they wrote letters and read letters and gathered personal effects from the dying for the chaplain to mail home. They snipped locks of hair from the dead, accepted violet nosegays handed to them by marching troops, and offered their necklaces for luck. Their encouraging words helped men focus on what was positive: "If the right arm is missing, then learn to write with the left. If your legs are gone, learn to knit or carve; read to those who are blind." Always, nutrition was stressed to facilitate healing.

Slates, carving tools, flannel shirts, books, Bibles, and forty-eight Boston rocking chairs were donated to the Fairfax Hospital; time spent in the rocking chairs lifted the men's spirits tremendously. Fabric arrived from Ladies' Aid Societies to make slings. One batch of old-fashioned yellow-flowered cloth came with this feeble-handed note "This material was strong. It was all I had. I am old and poor and cannot do much." Very often the milkman could not deliver due to swollen rivers and storms, so condensed canned milk was a blessing.

Trains continuously arrived filled with wounded. In June 1863, seven hundred arrived at once. The fittest patients had to be discharged so the new patients could have beds. Many Civil War hospitals were not as well equipped as Jane's; other nurses reported meals served on newspapers: "a thick slab of bread holding a cold potato and a glob of fat." All these letters record how heartwrenching and draining this work was and how many men suffered slow, painful deaths. Hurried pages of soldiers' journals reflect the weariness of battle and camp sickness.

Later, after the war, chosen to serve as a leader at military hospitals in Rhode Island and Maryland, Jane insisted her nurses exhibit exemplary behavior. She donated her own wages back to the hospital for the soldiers' needs. Newly freed young black women were trained at her vocational schools, where they were taught to make clothes and do housework and needlework. Jane contributed and solicited scholarship money for this school and monitored its progress.

Perhaps her most impressive post, however, was as resident director of the newly formed Presbyterian Hospital of New York, to which she was appointed in 1872. There she instructed nurses, and her sister, Abby, organized the multilayered facility. Suffering from the effects of rheumatic fever, Jane had to resign her position at Presbyterian Hospital in 1876. Once an accomplished mariner who loved to sail her boat, *The Quakerness*, Jane was now an invalid. Abby cared for her until her death in 1891.

JANE STUART WOOLSEY, UNION NURSE FROM CAMP, NEAR ALEXANDRIA, 1862

Now are the wolf's bloodied cubs
piled in planked wagon beds
and blue grapes crushed.

Now are the skin of summer's trees
and the dust of peaches buttoned
shirts filled with empty sleeves.

Behold the pumice fog
and dingy bread of winter, earth
bent over, gagging on its wine.

This is the first crop
of cotton bodies, the gray sky's
appaloosa ponies begging apples.

Here is the clay returned,
the elephant falling into his trunk,
the mourning doves' black lace gloves.

NURSE'S LETTER, MAY 30, 1864, ARMORY SQUARE HOSPITAL, WASHINGTON, D.C.

Miss Helen Griggs, Union Nurse

My Dear Mrs. Metternich: I cannot write a connected letter; I lost my senses
two weeks ago and haven't known my own name for a week. I cannot begin to tell you of what we are going through. Miss Hill and Miss Akin say
the number of wounded after Chancellorsville was nothing; was mere play
to what this is. Oh! they are piled in on us till one's heart sinks, and I, who
am good in emergencies, energetic, and walk like seven men, slink to the
door of my ward and stand there, dreading to go in, feeling as if I were a
baby and that I would give a fortune to be well out of it. I know I have
utterly mistaken my calling, as I cannot get used to seeing the entire anatomy
of the human frame every time I turn around and am altogether demented.
Now don't you see by that sentence that I am? My only consolation is that
the other ladies all feel so too. Miss Merrill, whose mother is here; Miss

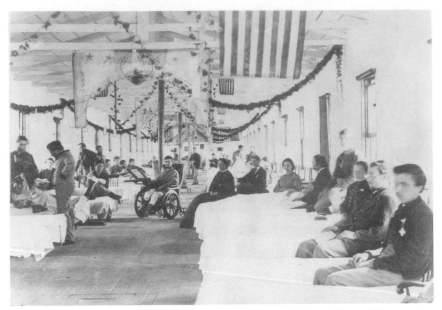

Armory Square Hospital, Washington, D. C., July 4, 1864. (Courtesy Library of Congress.)

Hill, a host herself; and Miss Akin all say and feel that their burden is greater than they can bear. I am glad for your sake you are not here; you could not stand it, even with those powders of Dr. Alcan. The odor is awful; the cases are all bad. I had forty-five dead today, two tents full beside the Dead House. The chapel is full of beds. We work hard, our beds are not made until we go down at "Taps." The care and confusion is immense—I am not exaggerating. My barrel of crackers and two huge boxes from New York have arrived. My brother at home sent me fifty dollars. I gave ten to Ward C in memory of its angel. Your Albert is doing fine. Pray for us. Helen

Rebecca Taylor

*M*iss Rebecca Taylor, one of the earliest head nurses of Massachusetts General Hospital in 1830, worked closely with and was respected by Dr. James Jackson. According to one of Dr. Jackson's colleagues, daily clinical dialogue between Nurse Taylor and Dr. Jackson was as spirited as any court room attorney's interrogation of a witness. In Dr. Jackson's letter to Anna Lowell in 1861, he describes Nurse Taylor as "quiet, with a dry-looking little body." Though she was small in stature, her works seem monumental. Dr. Jackson frequently asked the resident doctors their opinion regarding Nurse Taylor's knowledge and competency. The resident doctors always agreed "she was a fine nurse."

Elderly and ailing in 1860, Miss Rebecca Taylor retired from her nursing duties. The hospital board directive stated "her [Nurse Taylor's] hospital wages were to be continued." She became a patient in Massachusetts General, the institution she had served so faithfully for thirty-four years. Dr. Jackson's papers also noted Nurse Taylor had single-handedly cared for more than four thousand patients. Another colleague, Dr. Shaw, wrote her praises, saying, "her gentle manners and truly Christian life has won our gratitude and affection."

Thirteen years after Nurse Taylor's retirement in 1873, the Boston Training School for Nurses was in its embryonic stage of development. Physicians and

Miss Rebecca Taylor, age 68, December 4, 1860. From Dr. Henry Ingersoll Bowditch's album, Boston, Massachusetts. (Courtesy Francis A. Countway Library of Medicine, Harvard Medical Library.)

community leaders had envisioned the need for such an institution for more than twenty years. The lives of nurses in Boston before the days of formal training mirrored that of servants. Shift work lasted sixteen hours, and exhausted nurses slept on foldout cots stored in rooms between the wards. The nurses' small sleeping quarters were utilized by the medical staff during the day for consults and minor surgeries.

The Boston nurses in the early 1800s came from diverse socioeconomic backgrounds, age groups, and levels of intelligence and integrity. Their days were filled with carrying food on heavy trays; washing patients and dishes, linens and bandages; mending and pressing hospital laundry; followed by dusting and sweeping. For all the above, they were paid $7.50 a month. As medicine advanced, so did nursing, and while many physicians resisted upgrading this occupation, nursing evolved into a profession.

A TRIBUTE TO MISS REBECCA TAYLOR UPON RETIREMENT
AFTER THIRTY-FOUR YEARS

found poem by Dr. James Jackson, Massachusetts General, Boston, 1861

There is not any comparison
to be made between our good nurse
and Miss Nightingale.

The latter is a lady of education
and in a different rank of life.
My friend is one of much humbler pretensions.

She has been a hired nurse.
She sought employment for her living.
Having gained an appointment, she gave

herself to her duties. I have known
many good nurses in private families.
It is harder to perform faithfully and well

the nursing in a hospital.
I describe one of the most uniformly faithful,
fulfilling all her duties in a faultless manner.

I cannot help hoping that it will be useful
to hold up such an example for imitation.
I wish to point out how high are the duties of a nurse;

and how justly they entitle one,
who performs them skillfully and kindly,
to the love and respect of mankind.

Edith Cavell

*I*n Swardeston, England, Edith Cavell lived a comfortable Victorian girlhood, enjoying ice skating and lawn tennis, walking and swimming. A visual artist, this dark-haired girl did pencil sketches and watercolors of wildflowers, leaves, and farmhouses. Her father, Parson Frederick Cavell, was her first teacher, and he insisted his children learn French. A good student, Edith attended three boarding schools, a local high school, and graduated from Clevedon University.

She became a governess first, serving English families and one in Brussels in this capacity until her father became ill in 1895, prompting her return to England. While caring for her father, Edith decided nursing was her life's calling. One year later, she applied and was accepted for the position of assistant nurse class II at the London Fever Hospital. Here she would spend the next four years and four months learning the theory and practice of nursing. While in training, she received the Maidstone Medal with others in the nursing community for serving so tirelessly in the typhoid epidemic of 1897. For a time, she worked in the coal-mining district of Manchester and was known as "the Poor Man's Nightingale."

In 1907 a leading European surgeon, Dr. Depage, offered Edith the post of head matron to the nurses at the Rue de la Culture Clinique in Brussels. He needed a nursing leader with a firm hand and excellent command of the French language. Edith accepted the position at a salary of fifty pounds a year for over-

Edith Cavell, ca. 1901. (Courtesy Library of Congress.)

seeing all hospital departments and directing the newly established school of nursing. Her letters reflect an eagerness to meet such a challenge.

War came to Belgium in 1914, and Germany occupied this neutral country. Newspapers ceased to exist; coal loaded on railcars didn't move; food supplies dwindled; the ancient university town of Louvain was burned, its library gutted. When word came of the civilian massacre at Dinant, one of Edith's nurses walked the fifty kilometers and found the horrible rumors true: 612 bodies lay slaughtered.

In the fall of 1914 Edith agreed to care for and house two wounded English officers. This action was the beginning of her underground activities to help French and English soldiers get back to their battalions and Belgians to join the Allies. She hid soldiers in secret passageways, in outhouses, in apple barrels and with local families. Surviving letters and witness accounts credit Nurse Cavell with assisting between two hundred and four hundred soldiers, until her arrest in 1915. Of the hundreds of letters she wrote, eighteen survive. Moments before the Germans marched her out of the clinic, she burned many documents. Fifty years after her death by firing squad on October 12, 1915, a housekeeper found several diary entries sewn inside one of her final possessions, a cushion. For years, her mother received letters from soldiers who survived because of Nurse Cavell's efforts. One of these men instructed his family, "When I die, I'm to be buried in the hospital shirt given to me by Edith Cavell." In 1946, his family carried out his wish.

HOUSES ARE BURNING: BELGIUM, 1915

Edith Cavell, World War I nurse, executed

Write it on plain paper; use a pencil.
Three officers burst into my class,
and when they bound my hands,
my students screamed. Tell that the soldiers were German,
they marched me to a cell, smaller than father's
study, walls, dirty mule brown. There was a blanket,
a basin, a window the size of my family's Bible
in Norfolkshire. Tell them it was August, summer
worn out in a wrinkled skirt, and I was English.
In the margins, scribble, *She spoke no German.*

Do you believe history counts houses burned?
Lives lost? Then write my mother's name, Louise,

and say her geraniums and ivy bloomed in crocks
by the rock garden. Remember to say my father
was a minister and he wanted my sister and me to be
apostles, pull a ship full of hungry faces across
the water, so we became nurses. Belgium asked me
to train their nurses, and I wanted to teach.

People were being killed. Write it.
And write how we built a hospital, one hundred
seventy-five beds. Tell how soldiers came and died.
My nurses tended them like wrens nesting in a thunder-
storm. The armless were shaved, the wounded dressed.
My nurses were young and wore sadness like ribbons
in their hair. Write about the orphan ward,
how I would go there every night, alone, for one hour,
lift the most restless, hum lullabies I'd heard
above my pram. Write about England, my country,
filled with coal mines and poets in unmarked graves.

Write this. Soldiers took my white apron and blue dress,
handed me old trousers and a shirt. I rinsed my bloomers
out after my evening meal with what was left of my drinking
water. The soldiers never reached for my breast;
they spoke softly.
Write about the boy-guard who walked stiff-legged,
had a draining wound. Tell how I bandaged him
and he gave me soap. He might have been my son.

Write it down. Get it all down, how a man came
to our hospital; his eyes begged like a squirrel
caught in a steel trap. He said Germans would not
suspect a nurse, Belgium was neutral, the Allies
needed men. I agreed to help, hid soldiers and men
in our hospital, at night, we ran through narrow
streets like rats in a sewer, there was a tree
in the woods, I whistled the signal. Later,
once or twice, letters arrived.

Do you believe blood turns a stream red?
Then write this. I cut my hair with broken glass
and drew a calendar on the wall. Late September,

my bloomers glazed with frost. One morning the prison
chaplain visited, told me my nurses drafted a petition
for my release. They risked their lives by signing.
They were young and wore hope like a locket around
their necks. Get more paper.

Write about my trial. There was an interpreter
because I could not speak German, and thirty-five
of us were tried in two days. My barrister told me
there would be time for appeals. He spoke French,
a language I learned as a girl. French sounds like
the brook on my grandmother's farm, china cups
in mother's kitchen. Tell them I had hope
and read silence like scripture.

Write how soldiers stood by the chaplain
the last afternoon when he said my sentence was death
and would surely be appealed. We prayed, took
communion; he left. Then, the boy-guard brought
lemon tea cake, hugged me, pointed to his leg's scar.
After ten weeks, I loved him, this boy, who might
have been my son. Tell them it was 1915 and people
were dying. We were chewing off our legs to get out
of a thing bigger than England or Belgium
or the careless sky spilling its every star.

Do you believe all this happened? Still happens?
Then write on. In darkness, they bandaged my eyes,
covered my head with a veil. Walking to the wall,
I noticed one limped. German words clawed the air
like a hoe's clack in the garden. Rifles coughed,
cleared their throats. Please write this.
The soldiers refused to fire. An officer's bullet
split me like an olive. I saw geraniums—red, red,
red—and mother's ivy blooming in crocks. I was English,
here to train nurses.

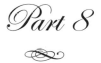

Part 8

Who knows what the body can remember
from far back, through the blood
traces of habit and sweat?
In a little while I'm going home.

Maggie Anderson,
"Abandoned Farm, Central Pennsylvania"

IF IT WEREN'T FOR EARS

Living where light is poor, sorting all day,
all night, the process is more complicated
for animals who live in air.

A telephone rings, your niece sounds
like your mother, a clock ticks above
her stove, steam hisses from a pot of beans.

Words are unclear, muddy, like your red boots
on her braided rug by the door slammed
to keep the cold wind outside.

Understanding all of this may be impossible
as you press a glass to the wall of memory's house,
for work done there was not much to look at,

no trumpet players, no violins, just warm
cornbread smell and lull of familiar voices
learning to signal one another, decoding

background noise, the separate yowls of hunger.
Temperature is important, in heat, a scream moves
faster, and sound is energy; once, scientists

increased volume so much laboratory mice
were burned—poor things—these ears,
dutiful guards to the brain's computer room.

They are the body's rain barrels for language,
the boxed ones, the pierced, the cauliflowered,
the ones joked about. Citizens compelled to listen

to lovers' lies, the embassy of golden pus, an alley
filled with neighborhood gossips, the editors
of truth, embalmers of lullabies, delicate

hammers for handling pressure, the bones
best protected, the ones who work together,
who create a sense of balance.

THE BRAIN'S SOLILOQUY

brain: from Webster's New Collegiate Dictionary

1a. *the portion of the vertebrate central nervous system that constitutes the organ of thought and neural coordination*

Say rather
I am the big city of the future
and a small town of the past,
a cauliflower who knows how
to wave a conductor's wand,
engine for a freight train
bearing a load of burning coals.

includes all the higher nervous centers receiving stimuli from the sense organs and interpreting and correlating them to formulate the motor impulses,

Say instead that I wore
a hard hat and was a harness
for the heart, my brilliance
was smiling like a village idiot
speaking a language
they couldn't understand
after my fevers and many explosions.

is made up of neurons and supporting nutritive structures,

As a girl, I fished
the brook of broken promises,
I was shy, carried old wood,
built this cache filled with provisions.
See, over there's
a backyard of nicknames
den of forgotten moments,
my collection of rocks
and fine ideas.

is enclosed within the skull, and is continuous with spinal cord through the foramen magnum.

Say I contain land
which is sparsely settled,
here, friends come and go,
their voices braid my seasons.
Say I was more
than a drawer of proverbs
or those pink messages never sent.
Tell them my name is genius.

CLAY PIGEON

I go to the bed where they have undressed him.
These common people move in a circle
around their son, who is a boy in a man's cobbled body.

His mother already in a wheelchair, on oxygen,
his father stooped and gray in a straw hat.
Call him love's surprise, love's accident,

a new planet come along in forty-three years,
a region of soft earth, free from pollution.
In our hospital gown, he becomes a choir boy,

a holy man smiling between his seizures.
Behold the dolphin she carried for nine months,
the brown bread they have baked and eaten together,

the hearth given to the chosen. Here is the son
who will never burst from the yellow school bus
waving his spelling test.

Here is the son who will never sing "Amazing Grace"
at Sunday's service. Here is the son who will never beg
the car keys for Saturday's game.

Here is the son who will never beat his wife
or snort cocaine. Behold the ground's brilliant root,
the stubborn movement of blood

through his body, the clay pigeon
others would shoot,
fearing his choking lullaby.

IN PRAISE OF HANDS

That they are slaves.
That each tendon's a rope
and the knuckles are pulleys.
That their white bones
line up like pieces of broken chalk.

They are bound by flesh
as leather around a Bible.
That they dance and write
in air the story
of what is lost, what is gained.

That they are soldiers
cut and bleeding, a link
to the heart's kingdom.
That they are so beautiful
a moon has landed on each finger.

That they are trained
for harps and hired for murder.
That the cuticles are shaped
like soft horseshoes.
They contain rivers.

That the ring finger's shyness
suffers when gripped by the powerful.
That the palm yields to blisters
and wears the calloused rags
of repetition.

That they are mythical
with their lifelines' hieroglyphics.
That they struggle
because of their great strength.
They are able to heal themselves.

That they know what it means
to draw the water
and work without pay.

That they will hide our eyes
and pray for our sins.

That they may lift the hammer
and lead our bodies to grace.
That they will make a print
like no other
until they wave goodbye.

Permissions

"Learning the Body" has a few phrases from Florence Nightingale's *Notes on Nursing* (New York: Dover, 1969). I am indebted to her skill as a writer and her wisdom as a caregiver.

"Standing There" is dedicated to Phyllis Fischer.

"Side Rails" is dedicated to Jerome J. Stanislaw, M.D., and his name is used with permission.

"Holding Back the World" first appeared as "Cotton" and is dedicated to Robert Stauter, M.D., friend and colleague, who lost his life on Swiss Air Flight 111.

"Letter to Christine: Girl Baby Found, Ohio Hospital, 1958" is a true story. All the names in this poem are used with permission.

Dr. Niemi's name is used with permission in "August Delivery."

"Hope Chest: What the Heart Teaches" is dedicated to my daughter, Summar.

"Letter to World War I Surgeon Dr. Henry Russell, from Nurse Jeanette Price, September 1929" has a story in it from World War I American Hospital Nurse, Ellen N. La Motte's book, *The Backwash of War* (New York: Putnam's, 1916). This book was banned and later republished. All nurses must be thankful for such an honest account of bedside care during such horrific conditions.

"After the Battle: In a Room Where We Have Tried to Save a Life" is dedicated to my nursing colleagues in the emergency room department of Forum Health Trumbull Memorial Hospital, Warren, Ohio.

"What Nurses Do: The Marriage of Suffering and Healing" uses a form similar to Alicia Ostriker's "Somalia" in the book *The Crack in Everything* (Pittsburgh: Univ. of Pittsburgh Press, 1996). I thank her for showing me how even the smallest person can speak through poetry.

"Interview With Sister Denis of St. Joseph's Hospitallers, Colony of Montreal, New France, 1694," uses a form similar to Muriel Rukeyser's "Statement, Phillipa Allen" from the book *The Collected Poems of Muriel Rukeyser* (New York: McGraw, 1978). I am indebted to her for showing me another technique for storytelling.

Most of the entries in "Wait for Morning: From Kate Cumming's Journal" are taken directly from her journal *Kate: The Journal of a Confederate Nurse* (Baton Rouge: Louisiana State Univ. Press, 1959). All nurses are indebted to her for her courage and for saving the story. I am also grateful to editor Richard Barksdale

Harwell and the Louisiana State University Press for reprinting the book and granting me permission to reprint some of Kate's moving journal entries.

In "A Tribute to Miss Rebecca Taylor upon Retirement after Thirty-four Years," Dr. James Jackson's letter excerpt had a few ellipses. I added nothing to this text but the line breaks. He was a founder of Massachusetts General Hospital.

To research the voice of political prisoners and write "Houses Are Burning, Belgium, 1915," I slowly read Carolyn Forché's heart-wrenching anthology *Against Forgetting* (New York: Norton, 1993). These poems comprise some of the most powerful testimony I've ever known. I thank Carolyn Forché for gathering the voices into one book, and I praise her for the fortitude to complete such a project.

"The Brain's Soliloquy" uses the dictionary form found in Lucille Clifton's "grandma we are poets." I am indebted to her for finding yet another form for poetry.

"In Praise of Hands" is dedicated to my partner, David.

Bibliography

Anderson, Maggie. *A Space Filled with Moving.* Pittsburgh: Univ. of Pittsburgh Press, 1992.

Austin, Anne L. *The Woolsey Sisters of New York.* Philadelphia: American Philosophical Society, 1971.

Billingsley, Andrew. *Climbing Jacob's Ladder: The Enduring Legacy of African American Families.* New York: Simon and Schuster, 1992.

Blair, John G. "Fall in 20.2 Inches With Flurries Due; 43 Dead Is Ohio Toll." *Cleveland Plain Dealer,* November 27, 1950.

Boland, Eavan. *Outside History.* New York: Norton, 1990.

Brande, Dorothea. *Becoming a Writer.* New York: Harcourt Brace, 1934.

Bryan, Sharon. "Where We Stand: Women Poets on Literary Tradition," *River City* 13, no. 2 (1993).

Burton, Katherine. *Sorrow Built a Bridge.* New York: Longmans, Green, 1937.

"City Battles Snow and Record Cold." *Cleveland Plain Dealer,* November 25, 1950.

Clifton, Lucille. "grandma, we are poets." In *Writing Poetry,* ed. Barbara Drake, 172–73. New York: Harcourt Brace, 1994.

Cumming, Kate. *Kate: The Journal of a Confederate Nurse.* Ed. Richard Barksdale Harwell. Baton Rouge: Louisiana State Univ. Press, 1959.

Dexter, Elisabeth A. *Career Women of America, 1776–1840.* Francestown, N.H.: Jones, 1968.

Dolan, Josephine. *The History of Nursing.* Philadelphia: W. B. Saunders, 1968.

Donahue, M. Patricia. *Nursing: The Finest Art.* St. Louis: Mosby, 1985.

Drake, Barbara. *Writing Poetry.* New York: Harcourt Brace, 1994.

Edelman, Helen Susan. "Safe to Talk: Abortion Narratives as a Rite of Return." *Journal of American Culture* 19 (1996): 29–39.

Ewers, Carolyn H. *Sidney Poitier: The Long Journey.* New York: Signet, 1969.

Farrow, John. *Damien the Leper.* New York: Doubleday, 1954.

Foran, J. K., and Sr. Helen Morrissey. *Jeanne Mance: Angel of the Colony.* Montreal: Herald, 1931.

Forché, Carolyn. *Against Forgetting.* New York: Norton, 1993.

Gibson, John M., and Mary S. Matthewson. *Three Centuries of Canadian Nursing.* Toronto: Macmillan, 1947.

Goldberg, Natalie. *Writing Down the Bones.* Boston: Shambhala, 1986.

Got, Ambroise. *The Case of Miss Cavell.* London: Hodder and Stoughton, 1921.

Grudin, Robert. *Time and the Art of Living.* New York: Ticknor and Fields, 1988.

Harjo, Joy. *She Had Some Horses.* New York: Thunder's Mouth, 1983.

Hobsbawn, Eric. *On History.* New York: New Press, 1997.

Jacobus, Mary. *Women Writing and Writing about Women.* New York: Barnes and Noble, 1979.

Kenny, Sister Elizabeth, and Martha Ostenso. *And They Shall Walk.* New York: Dodd, Mead, 1943.

Kumin, Maxine. *Our Ground Time Here Will Be Brief.* New York: Penguin, 1982.

Kunhardt, Philip B., Jr., ed. *Life: World War II.* Boston: Little, Brown, 1990.

La Motte, Ellen N. *The Backwash of War.* New York: Putnam's, 1916.

Lindsay, Mary, ed., and BrynWalls, art ed. *The Visual Dictionary of the Human Body.* New York: Kindersley, 1991.

Li Po. *The Works of Li Po the Chinese Poet.* Trans. Obata-Shigeyoshi. New York: Dutton, 1922.

Llewellyn, Chris. *Fragments from the Fire.* New York: Penguin, 1987.

Lorde, Audre. *The Cancer Journals.* San Francisco: Aunt Lute, 1980.

———. *The Marvelous Arithmetic of Distance.* New York: Norton, 1993.

Loveland, Roelif. "Heavy Snow Due Again Today; Six Dead Here; Guardsmen on Patrol." *Cleveland Plain Dealer,* November 26, 1950.

Millay, Edna St. Vincent. "Theme And Variations, 2." In *Love Poems by Women,* ed. Wendy Mulford. New York: Fawcett Columbine, 1990.

Neruda, Pablo. *The Captain's Verses.* Trans. Donald D. Walsh. New York: New Directions, 1972.

Nightingale, Florence. *Notes on Nursing: What It Is, What It Is Not.* 3d ed. New York: Dover, 1969.

Olsen, Tillie. *Silences.* New York: Dell, 1978.

Ostriker, Alicia Suskin. *The Crack in Everything.* Pittsburgh: Univ. of Pittsburgh Press, 1996.

"Poisonous Smog Like Donora's Kills 15 in Their Sleep in Mexico." *Cleveland Plain Dealer,* November 25, 1950.

Rukeyser, Muriel. *The Collected Poems of Muriel Rukeyser.* New York: McGraw-Hill, 1978.

Sexton, Anne. *Selected Poems of Anne Sexton.* Ed. Diane Wood Middlebrook and Diana Hume George. Boston: Houghton Mifflin, 1988.

Smith, W. Eugene. "Nurse Midwife Maude Callen Eases Pain of Birth, Life, and Death." *Life* 31, no. 23 (December 1951): 134–45.

Stearns, Amanda Akin. *The Lady Nurse of Ward E.* New York: Baker and Taylor, 1909.

Stoddard, Charles Warren. *The Lepers of Molokai.* Notre Dame, Ind.: Ave Maria Press, 1908.

Strickland, Thomas. *Hunter's Tropical Medicine.* Philadelphia: W. B. Saunders, 1984.

"Tanks, Trucks Rescue 54 Scouts Encamped in Metropolitan Parks." *Cleveland Plain Dealer,* November 27, 1950.

Thorndike, John. *Another Way Home: A Family's Journey through Mental Illness.* New York: Penguin, 1997.

Walker, Alice. *Anything We Love Can Be Saved.* New York: Random House, 1997.

Whitman, Walt. "Preface to *Leaves of Grass,* 1855." In *Walt Whitman's Poems,* ed. Gay Wilson Allen and Charles T. Davis. New York: New York Univ. Press, 1955.

X, Doctor. *Intern.* New York: Harper and Row, 1965.

Tenderly Lift Me
was designed and composed by Christine Brooks
in 10/13 Minion with display text in Edwardian Script;
printed by Thomson-Shore, Inc., of Dexter, Michigan;
and published by
The Kent State University Press
Kent, Ohio 44242 USA